Bariatric Surgery Journal

Acknowledgement

This journal is dedicated to you.

It's you who didn't take the easy way out.

It's you who made the decision to have Bariatric Surgery and therefore steer your life in a new direction.

Bariatric Surgery isn't magic. Because you have to work hard to get the results you want.

Redefine the next 8 weeks of your Bariatric Journey with your *Bariatric Surgery Journal*.

And even though Bariatric Surgery removes or bypasses 80% of your stomach - you're the one who is 100% committed to the lifestyle change you truly deserve.

This journal belongs to:

How to use this Journal

1 - Getting started
Journaling is a daily activity that you need to set time aside for. But it doesn't have to be a tedious task. Plan a few minutes every day to sit down and reflect on your daily activities and your bariatric goals.

2- Monthly, weekly and daily planners
This journal has 8 weeks worth of planners and trackers. Start with your monthly planner - there are 2 of them in the beginning of this journal - and continue to set your weekly goals. You can use the daily planners to maintain a clear overview of your daily activities including the bariatric goals you're working on. On top of that you can use the trackers which are included in the weekly pages, to keep yourself accountable throughout the week.

3- Self-reflection and brain dumps
This journal not only provides the opportunity to track your progress on and off the scale - it's also a tool to help you be more mindful. Add your self-reflective thoughts and anything that you want to write down to the self-reflection pages and the 'brain dump' notes.

4 - Take your time
Bariatric surgery is only the beginning of your journey and not your final destination. Changing your habits is hard work - and it takes time to learn how to stay consistent in doing so. Give yourself grace along the way. It's not about perfection, but about falling in love with the process of becoming the best version of yourself. You've got this!

Contents

Bariatric Surgery isn't about losing weight fast.

It's about creating habits that last.

My Bariatric Biography

About Me

Name: ....

Date of birth: ....

Favorite food pre-op: ....

Favorite food post-op: ....

About my Surgery

Type of surgery: ....

Surgery date: ....

Hospital/Clinic: ....

My surgeon's name: ....

My dietitian's name: ....

Key dates: ....

My Reasons Why

This is why I have Bariatric Surgery

1. ....
   ....

2. ....
   ....

3. ....
   ....

4. ....
   ....

5. ....
   ....

6. ....
   ....

My Reasons Why

This is why I have Bariatric Surgery

7. ....
....

8. ....
....

9. ....
....

10. ....
....

11. ....
....

12. ....
....

Bariatric Surgery
isn't the easy
way out.

It's just easy to
say it is.

Monthly Planner

Month: _____

MON	TUE	WED	THU	FRI	SAT	SUN

Priorities: _____

♡ ....
♡ ....
♡ ....
♡ ....
♡ ....

Notes:

To do: _____

☐ ....
☐ ....
☐ ....
☐ ....
☐ ....
☐ ....
☐ ....
☐ ....
☐ ....
☐ ....
☐ ....

6

Monthly Planner

Month: _____

MON	TUE	WED	THU	FRI	SAT	SUN

Priorities:

♡ ....

♡ ....

♡ ....

♡ ....

♡ ....

Notes:

To do:

☐ ....

☐ ....

☐ ....

☐ ....

☐ ....

☐ ....

☐ ....

☐ ....

☐ ....

☐ ....

☐ ....

☐ ....

Notes

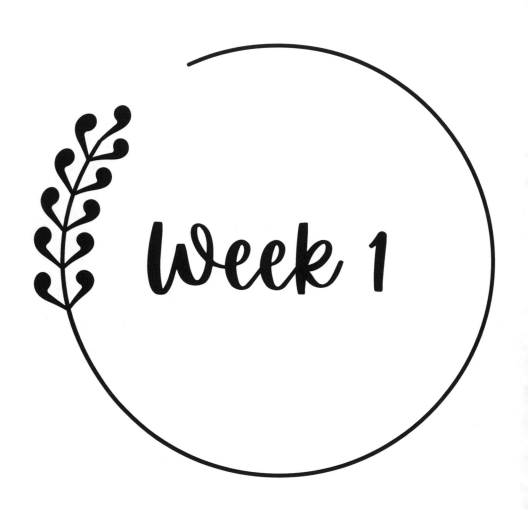

Week 1

Weekly Planner

Priorities:

♡ ....
♡ ....
♡ ....
♡ ....
♡ ....

To do:

☐ ....
☐ ....
☐ ....
☐ ....
☐ ....
☐ ....
☐ ....
☐ ....
☐ ....
☐ ....
☐ ....

Notes:

Monday

Tuesday

Wednesday

Thursday

Friday

Saturday

Sunday

Daily Planner

Daily tasks:

♡ ....
♡ ....
♡ ....
♡ ....
♡ ....

My mood:

☹ ☹ 😐 🙂 😄

Hours of sleep:

2	3	4	5	6	7	8	9	10	11	12
☐	☐	☐	☐	☐	☐	☐	☐	☐	☐	☐

Today's affirmation:

....

....

Notes:

Daily schedule:

Time	
8:00	
9:00	
10:00	
11:00	
12:00	
1:00	
2:00	
3:00	
4:00	
5:00	
6:00	
7:00	
8:00	
9:00	
10:00	

11

Food Diary

Breakfast

I ate because I felt:
- [ ] Hungry
- [ ] Tired
- [ ] Bored
- [ ] Emotional

Hunger/Fullness scale:

Ravenous ●●●●●○ Stuffed

Protein Carbs Sugar

Fat Calories Sodium

Lunch

I ate because I felt:
- [ ] Hungry
- [ ] Tired
- [ ] Bored
- [ ] Emotional

Hunger/Fullness scale:

Ravenous ●●●●●○ Stuffed

Protein Carbs Sugar

Fat Calories Sodium

Dinner

I ate because I felt:
- [ ] Hungry
- [ ] Tired
- [ ] Bored
- [ ] Emotional

Hunger/Fullness scale:

Ravenous ●●●●●○ Stuffed

Protein Carbs Sugar

Fat Calories Sodium

Snack 1

I ate because I felt:
- [ ] Hungry
- [ ] Tired
- [ ] Bored
- [ ] Emotional

Hunger/Fullness scale:

Ravenous ●●●●●○ Stuffed

Protein Carbs Sugar

Fat Calories Sodium

Snack 2

I ate because I felt:
- [ ] Hungry
- [ ] Tired
- [ ] Bored
- [ ] Emotional

Hunger/Fullness scale:

Ravenous ●●●●●○ Stuffed

Protein Carbs Sugar

Fat Calories Sodium

Snack 3

I ate because I felt:
- [ ] Hungry
- [ ] Tired
- [ ] Bored
- [ ] Emotional

Hunger/Fullness scale:

Ravenous ●●●●●○ Stuffed

Protein Carbs Sugar

Fat Calories Sodium

Vitamins: Yes! [ ]   I forgot... [ ]

12

Daily Planner

Tuesday

Daily tasks:

♡ ....
♡ ....
♡ ....
♡ ....
♡ ....

My mood:

☹ ☹ 😐 ☺ 😃

Hours of sleep:

2	3	4	5	6	7	8	9	10	11	12
☐	☐	☐	☐	☐	☐	☐	☐	☐	☐	☐

Today's affirmation:

....

....

Notes:

Daily schedule:

8.00	
9.00	
10.00	
11.00	
12.00	
1.00	
2.00	
3.00	
4.00	
5.00	
6.00	
7.00	
8.00	
9.00	
10.00	

13

Food Diary

Tuesday _____

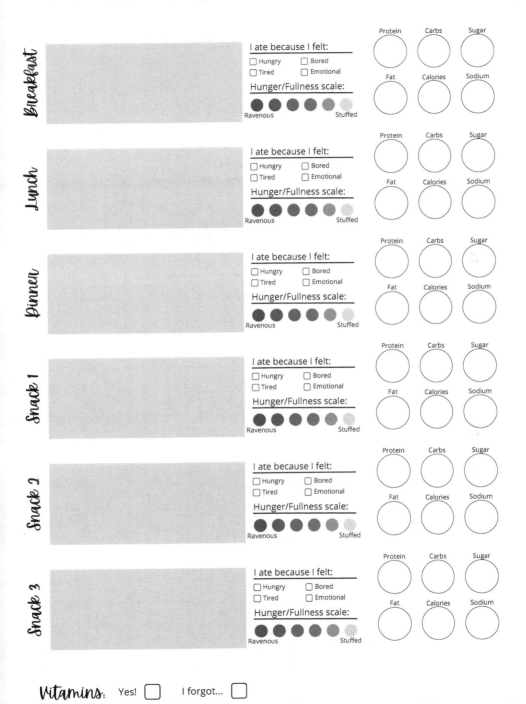

Breakfast

I ate because I felt:
- ☐ Hungry
- ☐ Tired
- ☐ Bored
- ☐ Emotional

Hunger/Fullness scale:

Ravenous ●●●●● Stuffed

Protein ○ Carbs ○ Sugar ○
Fat ○ Calories ○ Sodium ○

Lunch

I ate because I felt:
- ☐ Hungry
- ☐ Tired
- ☐ Bored
- ☐ Emotional

Hunger/Fullness scale:

Ravenous ●●●●● Stuffed

Protein ○ Carbs ○ Sugar ○
Fat ○ Calories ○ Sodium ○

Dinner

I ate because I felt:
- ☐ Hungry
- ☐ Tired
- ☐ Bored
- ☐ Emotional

Hunger/Fullness scale:

Ravenous ●●●●● Stuffed

Protein ○ Carbs ○ Sugar ○
Fat ○ Calories ○ Sodium ○

Snack 1

I ate because I felt:
- ☐ Hungry
- ☐ Tired
- ☐ Bored
- ☐ Emotional

Hunger/Fullness scale:

Ravenous ●●●●● Stuffed

Protein ○ Carbs ○ Sugar ○
Fat ○ Calories ○ Sodium ○

Snack 2

I ate because I felt:
- ☐ Hungry
- ☐ Tired
- ☐ Bored
- ☐ Emotional

Hunger/Fullness scale:

Ravenous ●●●●● Stuffed

Protein ○ Carbs ○ Sugar ○
Fat ○ Calories ○ Sodium ○

Snack 3

I ate because I felt:
- ☐ Hungry
- ☐ Tired
- ☐ Bored
- ☐ Emotional

Hunger/Fullness scale:

Ravenous ●●●●● Stuffed

Protein ○ Carbs ○ Sugar ○
Fat ○ Calories ○ Sodium ○

Vitamins: Yes! ☐   I forgot... ☐

14

Daily Planner

Daily tasks:

♡ ....
♡ ....
♡ ....
♡ ....
♡ ....

My mood:

😞 😟 😐 🙂 😃

Hours of sleep:

2	3	4	5	6	7	8	9	10	11	12
☐	☐	☐	☐	☐	☐	☐	☐	☐	☐	☐

Today's affirmation:

....

....

Notes:

Daily schedule:

Time	
8.00	
9.00	
10.00	
11.00	
12.00	
1.00	
2.00	
3.00	
4.00	
5.00	
6.00	
7.00	
8.00	
9.00	
10.00	

Food Diary

Breakfast

I ate because I felt:
- [ ] Hungry
- [ ] Tired
- [ ] Bored
- [ ] Emotional

Hunger/Fullness scale:

Ravenous ● ● ● ● ● ○ Stuffed

Protein ( ) Carbs ( ) Sugar ( )
Fat ( ) Calories ( ) Sodium ( )

Lunch

I ate because I felt:
- [ ] Hungry
- [ ] Tired
- [ ] Bored
- [ ] Emotional

Hunger/Fullness scale:

Ravenous ● ● ● ● ● ○ Stuffed

Protein ( ) Carbs ( ) Sugar ( )
Fat ( ) Calories ( ) Sodium ( )

Dinner

I ate because I felt:
- [ ] Hungry
- [ ] Tired
- [ ] Bored
- [ ] Emotional

Hunger/Fullness scale:

Ravenous ● ● ● ● ● ○ Stuffed

Protein ( ) Carbs ( ) Sugar ( )
Fat ( ) Calories ( ) Sodium ( )

Snack 1

I ate because I felt:
- [ ] Hungry
- [ ] Tired
- [ ] Bored
- [ ] Emotional

Hunger/Fullness scale:

Ravenous ● ● ● ● ● ○ Stuffed

Protein ( ) Carbs ( ) Sugar ( )
Fat ( ) Calories ( ) Sodium ( )

Snack 2

I ate because I felt:
- [ ] Hungry
- [ ] Tired
- [ ] Bored
- [ ] Emotional

Hunger/Fullness scale:

Ravenous ● ● ● ● ● ○ Stuffed

Protein ( ) Carbs ( ) Sugar ( )
Fat ( ) Calories ( ) Sodium ( )

Snack 3

I ate because I felt:
- [ ] Hungry
- [ ] Tired
- [ ] Bored
- [ ] Emotional

Hunger/Fullness scale:

Ravenous ● ● ● ● ● ○ Stuffed

Protein ( ) Carbs ( ) Sugar ( )
Fat ( ) Calories ( ) Sodium ( )

Vitamins: Yes! [ ]   I forgot... [ ]

Daily Planner

Daily tasks:

♡ ....
♡ ....
♡ ....
♡ ....
♡ ....

My mood:

☹ ☹ 😐 🙂 😀

Hours of sleep:

2	3	4	5	6	7	8	9	10	11	12
☐	☐	☐	☐	☐	☐	☐	☐	☐	☐	☐

Today's affirmation:

....

....

Notes:

Daily schedule:

8:00	
9:00	
10:00	
11:00	
12:00	
1:00	
2:00	
3:00	
4:00	
5:00	
6:00	
7:00	
8:00	
9:00	
10:00	

Food Diary

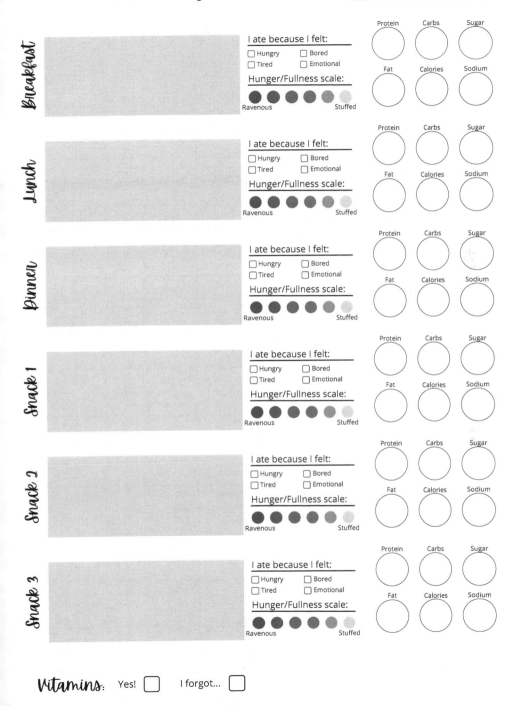

Breakfast

I ate because I felt:
- ☐ Hungry
- ☐ Tired
- ☐ Bored
- ☐ Emotional

Hunger/Fullness scale:
Ravenous ●●●●●● Stuffed

Protein · Carbs · Sugar · Fat · Calories · Sodium

Lunch

I ate because I felt:
- ☐ Hungry
- ☐ Tired
- ☐ Bored
- ☐ Emotional

Hunger/Fullness scale:
Ravenous ●●●●●● Stuffed

Protein · Carbs · Sugar · Fat · Calories · Sodium

Dinner

I ate because I felt:
- ☐ Hungry
- ☐ Tired
- ☐ Bored
- ☐ Emotional

Hunger/Fullness scale:
Ravenous ●●●●●● Stuffed

Protein · Carbs · Sugar · Fat · Calories · Sodium

Snack 1

I ate because I felt:
- ☐ Hungry
- ☐ Tired
- ☐ Bored
- ☐ Emotional

Hunger/Fullness scale:
Ravenous ●●●●●● Stuffed

Protein · Carbs · Sugar · Fat · Calories · Sodium

Snack 2

I ate because I felt:
- ☐ Hungry
- ☐ Tired
- ☐ Bored
- ☐ Emotional

Hunger/Fullness scale:
Ravenous ●●●●●● Stuffed

Protein · Carbs · Sugar · Fat · Calories · Sodium

Snack 3

I ate because I felt:
- ☐ Hungry
- ☐ Tired
- ☐ Bored
- ☐ Emotional

Hunger/Fullness scale:
Ravenous ●●●●●● Stuffed

Protein · Carbs · Sugar · Fat · Calories · Sodium

Vitamins: Yes! ☐   I forgot... ☐

Daily Planner

Friday

Daily tasks:

♡ ....
♡ ....
♡ ....
♡ ....
♡ ....

My mood:

☹ ☹ 😐 🙂 😄

Hours of sleep:

2 3 4 5 6 7 8 9 10 11 12
☐ ☐ ☐ ☐ ☐ ☐ ☐ ☐ ☐ ☐ ☐

Today's affirmation:

....

....

Notes:

Daily schedule:

8.00	
9.00	
10.00	
11.00	
12.00	
1.00	
2.00	
3.00	
4.00	
5.00	
6.00	
7.00	
8.00	
9.00	
10.00	

19

Food Diary

Friday _____

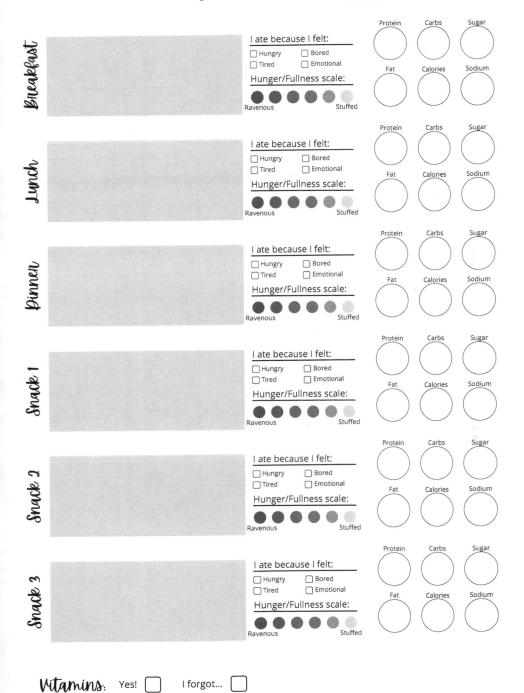

Breakfast

I ate because I felt:
- ☐ Hungry   ☐ Bored
- ☐ Tired   ☐ Emotional

Hunger/Fullness scale:

Ravenous ●●●●●○ Stuffed

Protein   Carbs   Sugar
Fat   Calories   Sodium

Lunch

I ate because I felt:
- ☐ Hungry   ☐ Bored
- ☐ Tired   ☐ Emotional

Hunger/Fullness scale:

Ravenous ●●●●●○ Stuffed

Protein   Carbs   Sugar
Fat   Calories   Sodium

Dinner

I ate because I felt:
- ☐ Hungry   ☐ Bored
- ☐ Tired   ☐ Emotional

Hunger/Fullness scale:

Ravenous ●●●●●○ Stuffed

Protein   Carbs   Sugar
Fat   Calories   Sodium

Snack 1

I ate because I felt:
- ☐ Hungry   ☐ Bored
- ☐ Tired   ☐ Emotional

Hunger/Fullness scale:

Ravenous ●●●●●○ Stuffed

Protein   Carbs   Sugar
Fat   Calories   Sodium

Snack 2

I ate because I felt:
- ☐ Hungry   ☐ Bored
- ☐ Tired   ☐ Emotional

Hunger/Fullness scale:

Ravenous ●●●●●○ Stuffed

Protein   Carbs   Sugar
Fat   Calories   Sodium

Snack 3

I ate because I felt:
- ☐ Hungry   ☐ Bored
- ☐ Tired   ☐ Emotional

Hunger/Fullness scale:

Ravenous ●●●●●○ Stuffed

Protein   Carbs   Sugar
Fat   Calories   Sodium

Vitamins: Yes! ☐   I forgot... ☐

Daily Planner

Daily tasks:

♡ ....
♡ ....
♡ ....
♡ ....
♡ ....

My mood:

☹ ☹ 😐 🙂 😄

Hours of sleep:

2	3	4	5	6	7	8	9	10	11	12
☐	☐	☐	☐	☐	☐	☐	☐	☐	☐	☐

Today's affirmation:

....

....

Notes:

Daily schedule:

8.00	
9.00	
10.00	
11.00	
12.00	
1.00	
2.00	
3.00	
4.00	
5.00	
6.00	
7.00	
8.00	
9.00	
10.00	

21

Food Diary

Breakfast

I ate because I felt:

- [ ] Hungry
- [ ] Tired
- [ ] Bored
- [ ] Emotional

Hunger/Fullness scale:

Ravenous ●●●●●○ Stuffed

Protein ○ Carbs ○ Sugar ○
Fat ○ Calories ○ Sodium ○

Lunch

I ate because I felt:

- [ ] Hungry
- [ ] Tired
- [ ] Bored
- [ ] Emotional

Hunger/Fullness scale:

Ravenous ●●●●●○ Stuffed

Protein ○ Carbs ○ Sugar ○
Fat ○ Calories ○ Sodium ○

Dinner

I ate because I felt:

- [ ] Hungry
- [ ] Tired
- [ ] Bored
- [ ] Emotional

Hunger/Fullness scale:

Ravenous ●●●●○○ Stuffed

Protein ○ Carbs ○ Sugar ○
Fat ○ Calories ○ Sodium ○

Snack 1

I ate because I felt:

- [ ] Hungry
- [ ] Tired
- [ ] Bored
- [ ] Emotional

Hunger/Fullness scale:

Ravenous ●●●●●○ Stuffed

Protein ○ Carbs ○ Sugar ○
Fat ○ Calories ○ Sodium ○

Snack 2

I ate because I felt:

- [ ] Hungry
- [ ] Tired
- [ ] Bored
- [ ] Emotional

Hunger/Fullness scale:

Ravenous ●●●●●○ Stuffed

Protein ○ Carbs ○ Sugar ○
Fat ○ Calories ○ Sodium ○

Snack 3

I ate because I felt:

- [ ] Hungry
- [ ] Tired
- [ ] Bored
- [ ] Emotional

Hunger/Fullness scale:

Ravenous ●●●●●○ Stuffed

Protein ○ Carbs ○ Sugar ○
Fat ○ Calories ○ Sodium ○

Vitamins: Yes! [ ]   I forgot... [ ]

Daily Planner

Daily tasks:

♡ ....
♡ ....
♡ ....
♡ ....
♡ ....

My mood:

☹ ☹ 😐 🙂 😄

Hours of sleep:

2	3	4	5	6	7	8	9	10	11	12
☐	☐	☐	☐	☐	☐	☐	☐	☐	☐	☐

Today's affirmation:

....

....

Notes:

Daily schedule:

8.00	
9.00	
10.00	
11.00	
12.00	
1.00	
2.00	
3.00	
4.00	
5.00	
6.00	
7.00	
8.00	
9.00	
10.00	

23

Food Diary

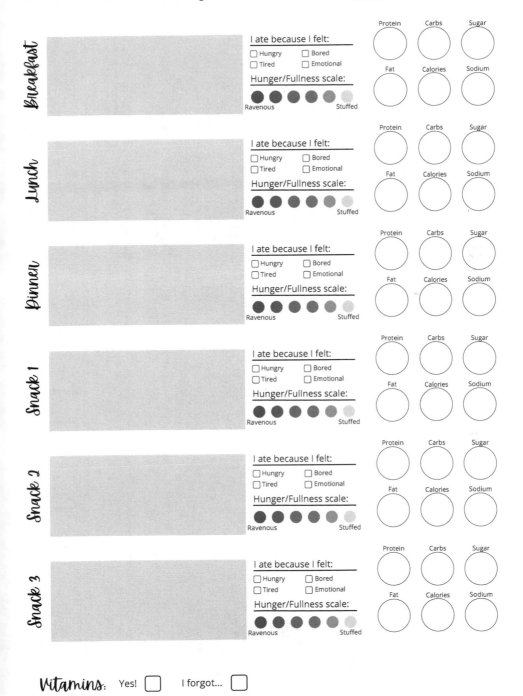

Breakfast

I ate because I felt:
- [ ] Hungry
- [ ] Bored
- [ ] Tired
- [ ] Emotional

Hunger/Fullness scale:

Ravenous — Stuffed

Protein | Carbs | Sugar
Fat | Calories | Sodium

Lunch

I ate because I felt:
- [ ] Hungry
- [ ] Bored
- [ ] Tired
- [ ] Emotional

Hunger/Fullness scale:

Ravenous — Stuffed

Protein | Carbs | Sugar
Fat | Calories | Sodium

Dinner

I ate because I felt:
- [ ] Hungry
- [ ] Bored
- [ ] Tired
- [ ] Emotional

Hunger/Fullness scale:

Ravenous — Stuffed

Protein | Carbs | Sugar
Fat | Calories | Sodium

Snack 1

I ate because I felt:
- [ ] Hungry
- [ ] Bored
- [ ] Tired
- [ ] Emotional

Hunger/Fullness scale:

Ravenous — Stuffed

Protein | Carbs | Sugar
Fat | Calories | Sodium

Snack 2

I ate because I felt:
- [ ] Hungry
- [ ] Bored
- [ ] Tired
- [ ] Emotional

Hunger/Fullness scale:

Ravenous — Stuffed

Protein | Carbs | Sugar
Fat | Calories | Sodium

Snack 3

I ate because I felt:
- [ ] Hungry
- [ ] Bored
- [ ] Tired
- [ ] Emotional

Hunger/Fullness scale:

Ravenous — Stuffed

Protein | Carbs | Sugar
Fat | Calories | Sodium

Vitamins: Yes! [ ]   I forgot... [ ]

Hydration Tracker

Week 1 _____

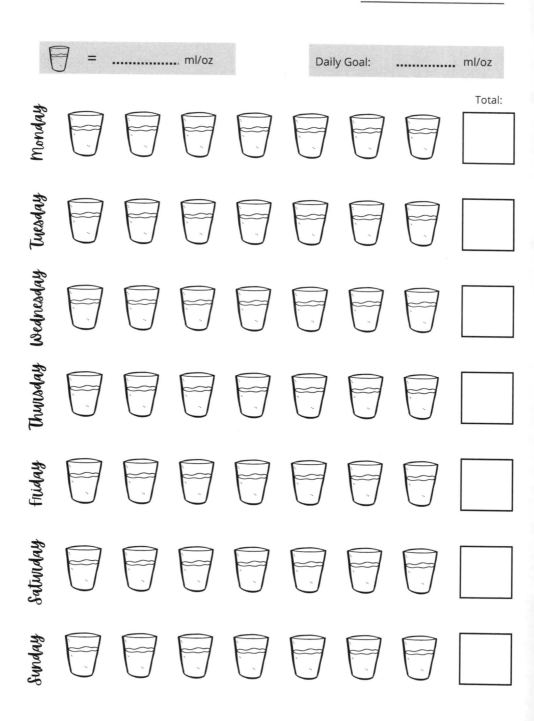

🥛 = ... ml/oz   Daily Goal: .... ml/oz

Monday   Total:

Tuesday

Wednesday

Thursday

Friday

Saturday

Sunday

Meal Planner

Week 1

Meals:

Grocery List:

Monday

Tuesday

Wednesday

Thursday

Friday

Saturday

Sunday

♡ ....
♡ ....
♡ ....
♡ ....
♡ ....
♡ ....
♡ ....
♡ ....
♡ ....
♡ ....
♡ ....
♡ ....
♡ ....
♡ ....
♡ ....
♡ ....
♡ ....
♡ ....
♡ ....
♡ ....
♡ ....
♡ ....
♡ ....

Activity Tracker

Week 1

Daily Target: .... minutes

Monday

Minutes:

Tuesday

Wednesday

Thursday

Friday

Saturday

Sunday

Habit Tracker

Habit	MON	TUE	WED	THU	FRI	SAT	SUN
	○	○	○	○	○	○	○
	○	○	○	○	○	○	○
	○	○	○	○	○	○	○
	○	○	○	○	○	○	○
	○	○	○	○	○	○	○
	○	○	○	○	○	○	○
	○	○	○	○	○	○	○
	○	○	○	○	○	○	○
	○	○	○	○	○	○	○
	○	○	○	○	○	○	○
	○	○	○	○	○	○	○
	○	○	○	○	○	○	○
	○	○	○	○	○	○	○
	○	○	○	○	○	○	○
	○	○	○	○	○	○	○
	○	○	○	○	○	○	○
	○	○	○	○	○	○	○

Notes:

Bariatric Surgery resized your stomach.

But it's in your hands to make things work.

Weigh-In

Highest Weight

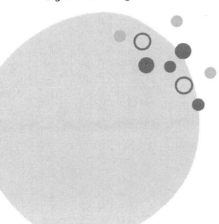

Weight Last Week

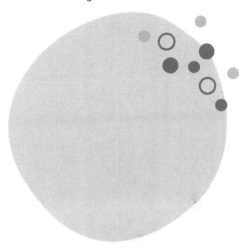

Weekly Weight Loss +/-

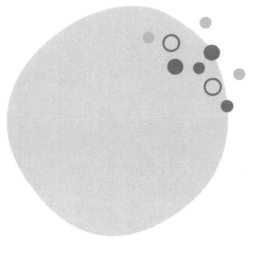

Current Weight

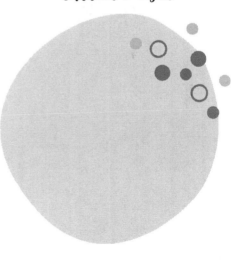

Notes:

....

....

Measurements

	Highest	Last Week	This Week	Lost
Neck				
Shoulders				
Chest				
Right Arm				
Left Arm				
Waist				
Hips				
Right Thigh				
Left Thigh				
Right Calf				
Left Calf				

Notes:

....

....

....

Progress Picture

Worthy Then

Worthy Now

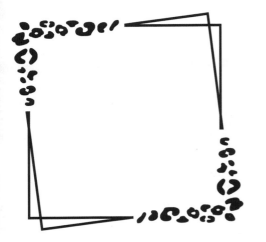

Date: ....

Weight: ....

Date: ....

Weight: ....

Describe how you felt in both pictures:

....

....

....

....

Reflection

Skills I have worked on this week:

I still need to be more mindful of:

I am thankful for:

Next week I will focus more on:

Brain Dump

Week 1

What's on your mind?

....

....

....

....

....

....

....

....

....

....

....

....

....

....

....

....

....

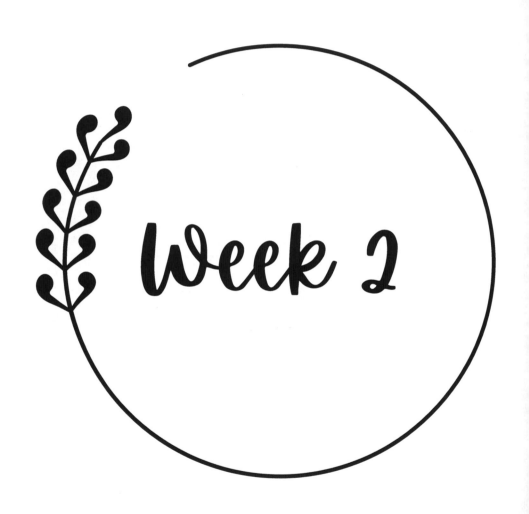

Week 2

Weekly Planner

Priorities:

♡ ....
♡ ....
♡ ....
♡ ....
♡ ....

To do:

☐ ....
☐ ....
☐ ....
☐ ....
☐ ....
☐ ....
☐ ....
☐ ....
☐ ....
☐ ....
☐ ....

Notes:

Monday

Tuesday

Wednesday

Thursday

Friday

Saturday

Sunday

Daily Planner

Daily tasks:

♡ ....
♡ ....
♡ ....
♡ ....
♡ ....

My mood:

☹ ☹ 😐 🙂 😃

Hours of sleep:

2 3 4 5 6 7 8 9 10 11 12
☐ ☐ ☐ ☐ ☐ ☐ ☐ ☐ ☐ ☐ ☐

Today's affirmation:

....
....

Notes:

Daily schedule:

8:00	
9:00	
10:00	
11:00	
12:00	
1:00	
2:00	
3:00	
4:00	
5:00	
6:00	
7:00	
8:00	
9:00	
10:00	

37

Food Diary

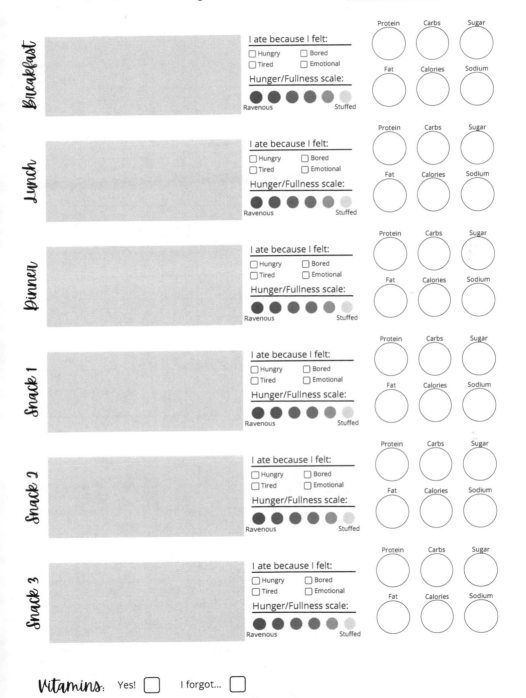

Breakfast

I ate because I felt:
- ☐ Hungry
- ☐ Tired
- ☐ Bored
- ☐ Emotional

Hunger/Fullness scale:

Ravenous ●●●●● Stuffed

Protein ○ Carbs ○ Sugar ○

Fat ○ Calories ○ Sodium ○

Lunch

I ate because I felt:
- ☐ Hungry
- ☐ Tired
- ☐ Bored
- ☐ Emotional

Hunger/Fullness scale:

Ravenous ●●●●● Stuffed

Protein ○ Carbs ○ Sugar ○

Fat ○ Calories ○ Sodium ○

Dinner

I ate because I felt:
- ☐ Hungry
- ☐ Tired
- ☐ Bored
- ☐ Emotional

Hunger/Fullness scale:

Ravenous ●●●●● Stuffed

Protein ○ Carbs ○ Sugar ○

Fat ○ Calories ○ Sodium ○

Snack 1

I ate because I felt:
- ☐ Hungry
- ☐ Tired
- ☐ Bored
- ☐ Emotional

Hunger/Fullness scale:

Ravenous ●●●●● Stuffed

Protein ○ Carbs ○ Sugar ○

Fat ○ Calories ○ Sodium ○

Snack 2

I ate because I felt:
- ☐ Hungry
- ☐ Tired
- ☐ Bored
- ☐ Emotional

Hunger/Fullness scale:

Ravenous ●●●●● Stuffed

Protein ○ Carbs ○ Sugar ○

Fat ○ Calories ○ Sodium ○

Snack 3

I ate because I felt:
- ☐ Hungry
- ☐ Tired
- ☐ Bored
- ☐ Emotional

Hunger/Fullness scale:

Ravenous ●●●●● Stuffed

Protein ○ Carbs ○ Sugar ○

Fat ○ Calories ○ Sodium ○

Vitamins: Yes! ☐   I forgot... ☐

38

Daily Planner

Daily tasks:

- ♡ ....
- ♡ ....
- ♡ ....
- ♡ ....
- ♡ ....

My mood:

☹ ☹ 😐 🙂 😄

Hours of sleep:

2	3	4	5	6	7	8	9	10	11	12
☐	☐	☐	☐	☐	☐	☐	☐	☐	☐	☐

Today's affirmation:

....

....

Notes:

Daily schedule:

8.00	
9.00	
10.00	
11.00	
12.00	
1.00	
2.00	
3.00	
4.00	
5.00	
6.00	
7.00	
8.00	
9.00	
10.00	

Food Diary

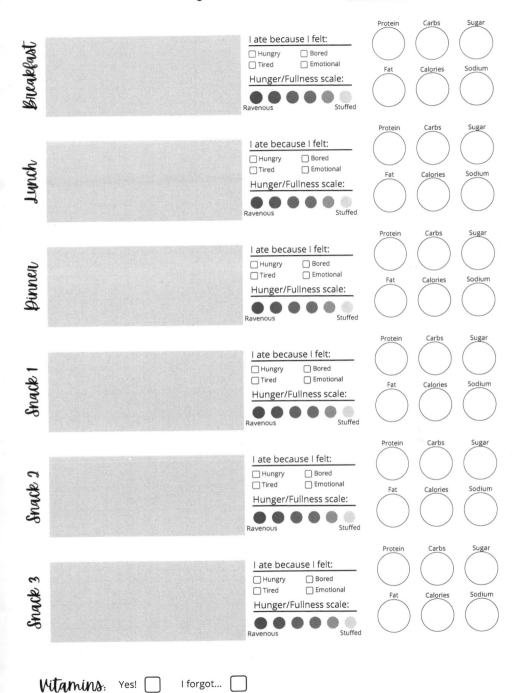

Tuesday _____

Breakfast

I ate because I felt:
- ☐ Hungry
- ☐ Tired
- ☐ Bored
- ☐ Emotional

Hunger/Fullness scale:
Ravenous ●●●●● Stuffed

Protein · Carbs · Sugar
Fat · Calories · Sodium

Lunch

I ate because I felt:
- ☐ Hungry
- ☐ Tired
- ☐ Bored
- ☐ Emotional

Hunger/Fullness scale:
Ravenous ●●●●● Stuffed

Protein · Carbs · Sugar
Fat · Calories · Sodium

Dinner

I ate because I felt:
- ☐ Hungry
- ☐ Tired
- ☐ Bored
- ☐ Emotional

Hunger/Fullness scale:
Ravenous ●●●●● Stuffed

Protein · Carbs · Sugar
Fat · Calories · Sodium

Snack 1

I ate because I felt:
- ☐ Hungry
- ☐ Tired
- ☐ Bored
- ☐ Emotional

Hunger/Fullness scale:
Ravenous ●●●●● Stuffed

Protein · Carbs · Sugar
Fat · Calories · Sodium

Snack 2

I ate because I felt:
- ☐ Hungry
- ☐ Tired
- ☐ Bored
- ☐ Emotional

Hunger/Fullness scale:
Ravenous ●●●●● Stuffed

Protein · Carbs · Sugar
Fat · Calories · Sodium

Snack 3

I ate because I felt:
- ☐ Hungry
- ☐ Tired
- ☐ Bored
- ☐ Emotional

Hunger/Fullness scale:
Ravenous ●●●●● Stuffed

Protein · Carbs · Sugar
Fat · Calories · Sodium

Vitamins: Yes! ☐   I forgot... ☐

Daily Planner

Wednesday

Daily tasks:

♡ ....
♡ ....
♡ ....
♡ ....
♡ ....

My mood:

☹ ☹ 😐 ☺ 😃

Hours of sleep:

2	3	4	5	6	7	8	9	10	11	12
☐	☐	☐	☐	☐	☐	☐	☐	☐	☐	☐

Today's affirmation:

....

....

Notes:

Daily schedule:

8:00	
9:00	
10:00	
11:00	
12:00	
1:00	
2:00	
3:00	
4:00	
5:00	
6:00	
7:00	
8:00	
9:00	
10:00	

Food Diary

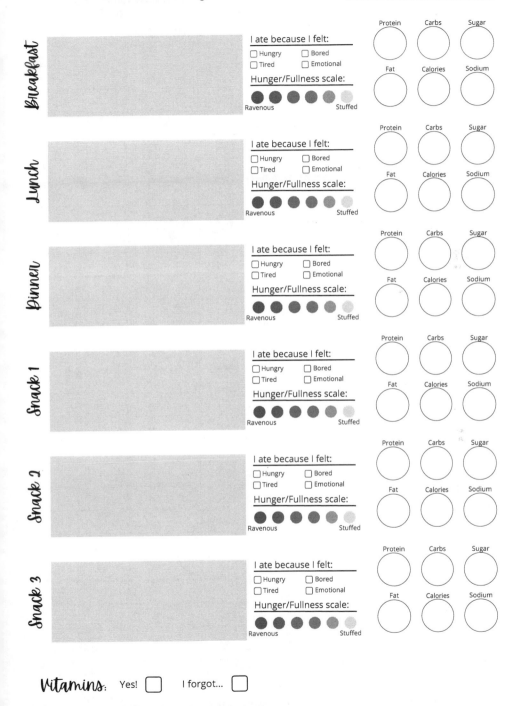

Breakfast

I ate because I felt:
- [ ] Hungry
- [ ] Tired
- [ ] Bored
- [ ] Emotional

Hunger/Fullness scale:

Ravenous — Stuffed

Protein | Carbs | Sugar
Fat | Calories | Sodium

Lunch

I ate because I felt:
- [ ] Hungry
- [ ] Tired
- [ ] Bored
- [ ] Emotional

Hunger/Fullness scale:

Ravenous — Stuffed

Protein | Carbs | Sugar
Fat | Calories | Sodium

Dinner

I ate because I felt:
- [ ] Hungry
- [ ] Tired
- [ ] Bored
- [ ] Emotional

Hunger/Fullness scale:

Ravenous — Stuffed

Protein | Carbs | Sugar
Fat | Calories | Sodium

Snack 1

I ate because I felt:
- [ ] Hungry
- [ ] Tired
- [ ] Bored
- [ ] Emotional

Hunger/Fullness scale:

Ravenous — Stuffed

Protein | Carbs | Sugar
Fat | Calories | Sodium

Snack 2

I ate because I felt:
- [ ] Hungry
- [ ] Tired
- [ ] Bored
- [ ] Emotional

Hunger/Fullness scale:

Ravenous — Stuffed

Protein | Carbs | Sugar
Fat | Calories | Sodium

Snack 3

I ate because I felt:
- [ ] Hungry
- [ ] Tired
- [ ] Bored
- [ ] Emotional

Hunger/Fullness scale:

Ravenous — Stuffed

Protein | Carbs | Sugar
Fat | Calories | Sodium

Vitamins: Yes! [ ]   I forgot... [ ]

Daily Planner

Thursday

Daily tasks:

♡ ....
♡ ....
♡ ....
♡ ....
♡ ....

My mood:

☹ ☹ 😐 🙂 😀

Hours of sleep:

2	3	4	5	6	7	8	9	10	11	12
☐	☐	☐	☐	☐	☐	☐	☐	☐	☐	☐

Today's affirmation:

....

....

Notes:

Daily schedule:

8.00	
9.00	
10.00	
11.00	
12.00	
1.00	
2.00	
3.00	
4.00	
5.00	
6.00	
7.00	
8.00	
9.00	
10.00	

Food Diary

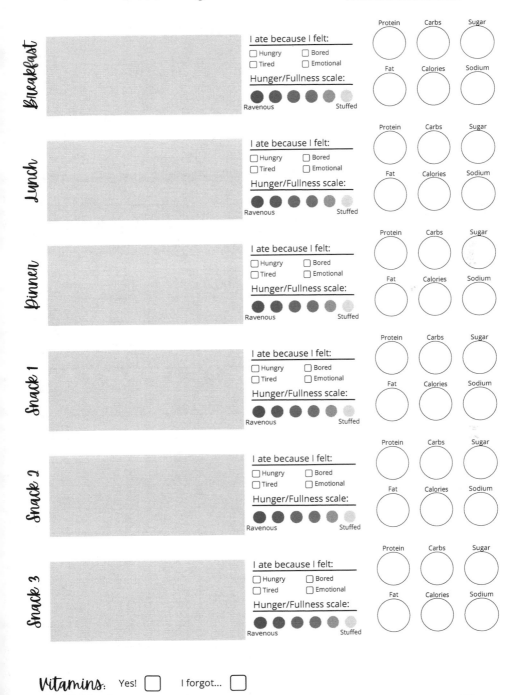

Breakfast

I ate because I felt:
- [ ] Hungry
- [ ] Tired
- [ ] Bored
- [ ] Emotional

Hunger/Fullness scale:
Ravenous ●●●●● Stuffed

Protein Carbs Sugar
Fat Calories Sodium

Lunch

I ate because I felt:
- [ ] Hungry
- [ ] Tired
- [ ] Bored
- [ ] Emotional

Hunger/Fullness scale:
Ravenous ●●●●● Stuffed

Protein Carbs Sugar
Fat Calories Sodium

Dinner

I ate because I felt:
- [ ] Hungry
- [ ] Tired
- [ ] Bored
- [ ] Emotional

Hunger/Fullness scale:
Ravenous ●●●●● Stuffed

Protein Carbs Sugar
Fat Calories Sodium

Snack 1

I ate because I felt:
- [ ] Hungry
- [ ] Tired
- [ ] Bored
- [ ] Emotional

Hunger/Fullness scale:
Ravenous ●●●●● Stuffed

Protein Carbs Sugar
Fat Calories Sodium

Snack 2

I ate because I felt:
- [ ] Hungry
- [ ] Tired
- [ ] Bored
- [ ] Emotional

Hunger/Fullness scale:
Ravenous ●●●●● Stuffed

Protein Carbs Sugar
Fat Calories Sodium

Snack 3

I ate because I felt:
- [ ] Hungry
- [ ] Tired
- [ ] Bored
- [ ] Emotional

Hunger/Fullness scale:
Ravenous ●●●●● Stuffed

Protein Carbs Sugar
Fat Calories Sodium

Vitamins: Yes! [ ]   I forgot... [ ]

Daily Planner

Daily tasks:

♡ ....
♡ ....
♡ ....
♡ ....
♡ ....

My mood:

😢 😦 😐 🙂 😄

Hours of sleep:

2	3	4	5	6	7	8	9	10	11	12
☐	☐	☐	☐	☐	☐	☐	☐	☐	☐	☐

Today's affirmation:

....

....

Notes:

Daily schedule:

8.00	
9.00	
10.00	
11.00	
12.00	
1.00	
2.00	
3.00	
4.00	
5.00	
6.00	
7.00	
8.00	
9.00	
10.00	

Food Diary

Breakfast

I ate because I felt:

- [ ] Hungry
- [ ] Tired
- [ ] Bored
- [ ] Emotional

Hunger/Fullness scale:

Ravenous ●●●●● Stuffed

Protein   Carbs   Sugar
Fat   Calories   Sodium

Lunch

I ate because I felt:

- [ ] Hungry
- [ ] Tired
- [ ] Bored
- [ ] Emotional

Hunger/Fullness scale:

Ravenous ●●●●● Stuffed

Protein   Carbs   Sugar
Fat   Calories   Sodium

Dinner

I ate because I felt:

- [ ] Hungry
- [ ] Tired
- [ ] Bored
- [ ] Emotional

Hunger/Fullness scale:

Ravenous ●●●●● Stuffed

Protein   Carbs   Sugar
Fat   Calories   Sodium

Snack 1

I ate because I felt:

- [ ] Hungry
- [ ] Tired
- [ ] Bored
- [ ] Emotional

Hunger/Fullness scale:

Ravenous ●●●●● Stuffed

Protein   Carbs   Sugar
Fat   Calories   Sodium

Snack 2

I ate because I felt:

- [ ] Hungry
- [ ] Tired
- [ ] Bored
- [ ] Emotional

Hunger/Fullness scale:

Ravenous ●●●●● Stuffed

Protein   Carbs   Sugar
Fat   Calories   Sodium

Snack 3

I ate because I felt:

- [ ] Hungry
- [ ] Tired
- [ ] Bored
- [ ] Emotional

Hunger/Fullness scale:

Ravenous ●●●●● Stuffed

Protein   Carbs   Sugar
Fat   Calories   Sodium

Vitamins: Yes! [ ]   I forgot... [ ]

Daily Planner

Daily tasks:

♡ ....
♡ ....
♡ ....
♡ ....
♡ ....

My mood:

☹ ☹ 😐 🙂 😄

Hours of sleep:

2	3	4	5	6	7	8	9	10	11	12
☐	☐	☐	☐	☐	☐	☐	☐	☐	☐	☐

Today's affirmation:

....

....

Notes:

Daily schedule:

8:00	
9:00	
10:00	
11:00	
12:00	
1:00	
2:00	
3:00	
4:00	
5:00	
6:00	
7:00	
8:00	
9:00	
10:00	

47

Food Diary

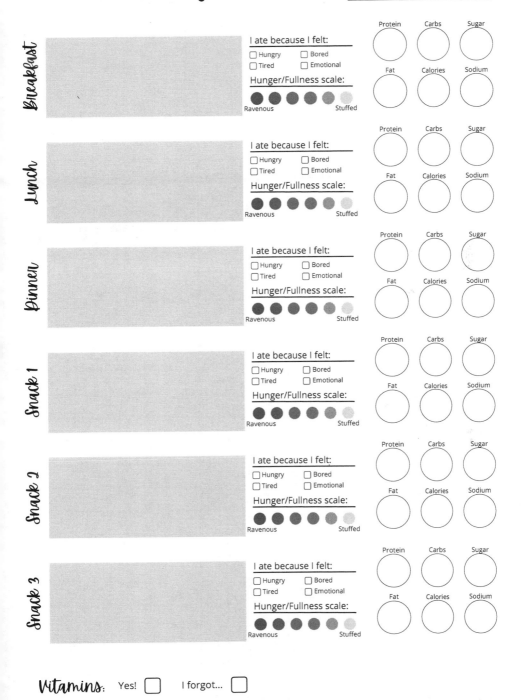

Saturday

Breakfast

I ate because I felt:
- ☐ Hungry
- ☐ Tired
- ☐ Bored
- ☐ Emotional

Hunger/Fullness scale:
Ravenous ●●●●●● Stuffed

Protein • Carbs • Sugar
Fat • Calories • Sodium

Lunch

I ate because I felt:
- ☐ Hungry
- ☐ Tired
- ☐ Bored
- ☐ Emotional

Hunger/Fullness scale:
Ravenous ●●●●●● Stuffed

Protein • Carbs • Sugar
Fat • Calories • Sodium

Dinner

I ate because I felt:
- ☐ Hungry
- ☐ Tired
- ☐ Bored
- ☐ Emotional

Hunger/Fullness scale:
Ravenous ●●●●●● Stuffed

Protein • Carbs • Sugar
Fat • Calories • Sodium

Snack 1

I ate because I felt:
- ☐ Hungry
- ☐ Tired
- ☐ Bored
- ☐ Emotional

Hunger/Fullness scale:
Ravenous ●●●●●● Stuffed

Protein • Carbs • Sugar
Fat • Calories • Sodium

Snack 2

I ate because I felt:
- ☐ Hungry
- ☐ Tired
- ☐ Bored
- ☐ Emotional

Hunger/Fullness scale:
Ravenous ●●●●●● Stuffed

Protein • Carbs • Sugar
Fat • Calories • Sodium

Snack 3

I ate because I felt:
- ☐ Hungry
- ☐ Tired
- ☐ Bored
- ☐ Emotional

Hunger/Fullness scale:
Ravenous ●●●●●● Stuffed

Protein • Carbs • Sugar
Fat • Calories • Sodium

Vitamins: Yes! ☐   I forgot... ☐

48

Daily Planner

Daily tasks:

♡ ....
♡ ....
♡ ....
♡ ....
♡ ....

My mood:

☹ ☹ 😐 ☺ 😄

Hours of sleep:

2	3	4	5	6	7	8	9	10	11	12
☐	☐	☐	☐	☐	☐	☐	☐	☐	☐	☐

Today's affirmation:

....
....

Notes:

Daily schedule:

8:00	
9:00	
10:00	
11:00	
12:00	
1:00	
2:00	
3:00	
4:00	
5:00	
6:00	
7:00	
8:00	
9:00	
10:00	

49

Food Diary

Breakfast

I ate because I felt:

- [ ] Hungry
- [ ] Tired
- [ ] Bored
- [ ] Emotional

Hunger/Fullness scale:

Ravenous ●●●●●● Stuffed

Protein · Carbs · Sugar

Fat · Calories · Sodium

Lunch

I ate because I felt:

- [ ] Hungry
- [ ] Tired
- [ ] Bored
- [ ] Emotional

Hunger/Fullness scale:

Ravenous ●●●●●● Stuffed

Protein · Carbs · Sugar

Fat · Calories · Sodium

Dinner

I ate because I felt:

- [ ] Hungry
- [ ] Tired
- [ ] Bored
- [ ] Emotional

Hunger/Fullness scale:

Ravenous ●●●●●● Stuffed

Protein · Carbs · Sugar

Fat · Calories · Sodium

Snack 1

I ate because I felt:

- [ ] Hungry
- [ ] Tired
- [ ] Bored
- [ ] Emotional

Hunger/Fullness scale:

Ravenous ●●●●●● Stuffed

Protein · Carbs · Sugar

Fat · Calories · Sodium

Snack 2

I ate because I felt:

- [ ] Hungry
- [ ] Tired
- [ ] Bored
- [ ] Emotional

Hunger/Fullness scale:

Ravenous ●●●●●● Stuffed

Protein · Carbs · Sugar

Fat · Calories · Sodium

Snack 3

I ate because I felt:

- [ ] Hungry
- [ ] Tired
- [ ] Bored
- [ ] Emotional

Hunger/Fullness scale:

Ravenous ●●●●●● Stuffed

Protein · Carbs · Sugar

Fat · Calories · Sodium

Vitamins: Yes! [ ]   I forgot... [ ]

Hydration Tracker Week 2

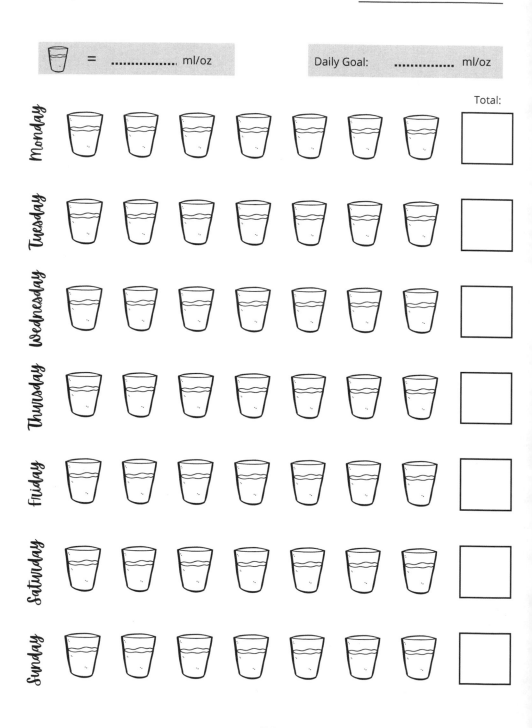

= .... ml/oz

Daily Goal: .... ml/oz

Total:

Monday

Tuesday

Wednesday

Thursday

Friday

Saturday

Sunday

Meal Planner

Meals:

Grocery List:

Monday

Tuesday

Wednesday

Thursday

friday

Saturday

Sunday

♡ ....
♡ ....
♡ ....
♡ ....
♡ ....
♡ ....
♡ ....
♡ ....
♡ ....
♡ ....
♡ ....
♡ ....
♡ ....
♡ ....
♡ ....
♡ ....
♡ ....
♡ ....
♡ ....
♡ ....
♡ ....
♡ ....
♡ ....
♡ ....

Activity Tracker

Daily Target: .... minutes

Minutes:

Monday

Tuesday

Wednesday

Thursday

Friday

Saturday

Sunday

Habit Tracker

Habit	MON	TUE	WED	THU	FRI	SAT	SUN
	○	○	○	○	○	○	○
	○	○	○	○	○	○	○
	○	○	○	○	○	○	○
	○	○	○	○	○	○	○
	○	○	○	○	○	○	○
	○	○	○	○	○	○	○
	○	○	○	○	○	○	○
	○	○	○	○	○	○	○
	○	○	○	○	○	○	○
	○	○	○	○	○	○	○
	○	○	○	○	○	○	○
	○	○	○	○	○	○	○
	○	○	○	○	○	○	○
	○	○	○	○	○	○	○
	○	○	○	○	○	○	○
	○	○	○	○	○	○	○
	○	○	○	○	○	○	○

Notes:

Just because it's called the 'honeymoon stage' doesn't mean that your first year post-op is going to be all sunshine and rainbows.

Weigh-In

Highest Weight

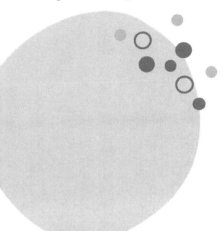

Weight Last Week

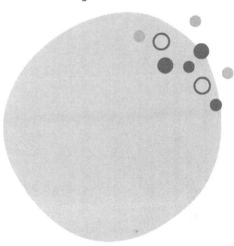

Weekly Weight Loss +/-

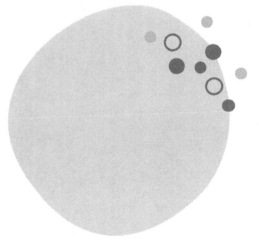

Current Weight

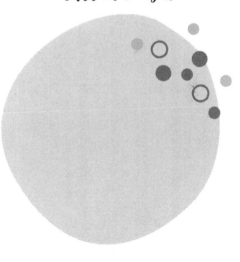

Notes:

....

....

Measurements

	Highest	Last Week	This Week	Lost
Neck				
Shoulders				
Chest				
Right Arm				
Left Arm				
Waist				
Hips				
Right Thigh				
Left Thigh				
Right Calf				
Left Calf				

Notes:

Progress Picture

Worthy Then   Worthy Now

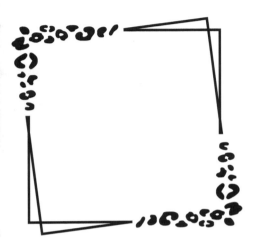
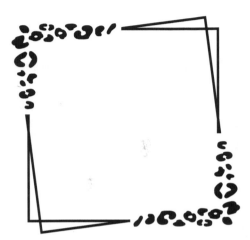

Date: ....   Date: ....

Weight: ....   Weight: ....

Describe how you felt in both pictures:

....

....

....

....

Reflection

Skills I have worked on this week:

....

....

....

....

I still need to be more mindful of:

....

....

....

....

I am thankful for:

....

....

....

....

Next week I will focus more on:

....

....

....

Brain Dump

What's on your mind?

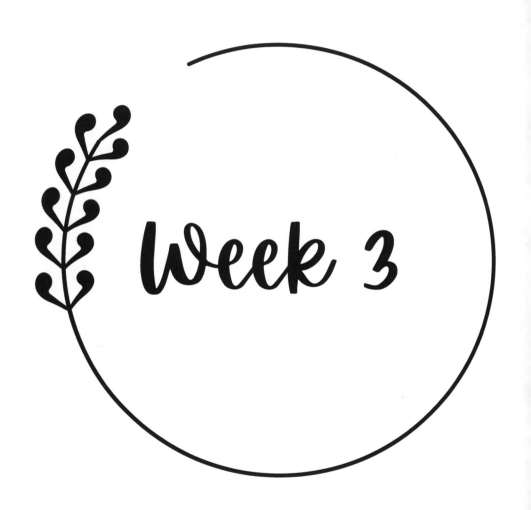

Week 3

Weekly Planner

Priorities:

♡ ....
♡ ....
♡ ....
♡ ....
♡ ....

To do:

☐ ....
☐ ....
☐ ....
☐ ....
☐ ....
☐ ....
☐ ....
☐ ....
☐ ....
☐ ....
☐ ....

Notes:

Monday

Tuesday

Wednesday

Thursday

Friday

Saturday

Sunday

Daily Planner

Daily tasks:

♡ ....
♡ ....
♡ ....
♡ ....
♡ ....

My mood:

☹ ☹ 😐 🙂 😃

Hours of sleep:

2	3	4	5	6	7	8	9	10	11	12
☐	☐	☐	☐	☐	☐	☐	☐	☐	☐	☐

Today's affirmation:

....
....

Notes:

Daily schedule:

8:00	
9:00	
10:00	
11:00	
12:00	
1:00	
2:00	
3:00	
4:00	
5:00	
6:00	
7:00	
8:00	
9:00	
10:00	

63

Food Diary

Breakfast

I ate because I felt:

- [ ] Hungry
- [ ] Tired
- [ ] Bored
- [ ] Emotional

Hunger/Fullness scale:

Ravenous ●●●●●● Stuffed

Protein ○ Carbs ○ Sugar ○
Fat ○ Calories ○ Sodium ○

Lunch

I ate because I felt:

- [ ] Hungry
- [ ] Tired
- [ ] Bored
- [ ] Emotional

Hunger/Fullness scale:

Ravenous ●●●●●● Stuffed

Protein ○ Carbs ○ Sugar ○
Fat ○ Calories ○ Sodium ○

Dinner

I ate because I felt:

- [ ] Hungry
- [ ] Tired
- [ ] Bored
- [ ] Emotional

Hunger/Fullness scale:

Ravenous ●●●●●● Stuffed

Protein ○ Carbs ○ Sugar ○
Fat ○ Calories ○ Sodium ○

Snack 1

I ate because I felt:

- [ ] Hungry
- [ ] Tired
- [ ] Bored
- [ ] Emotional

Hunger/Fullness scale:

Ravenous ●●●●●● Stuffed

Protein ○ Carbs ○ Sugar ○
Fat ○ Calories ○ Sodium ○

Snack 2

I ate because I felt:

- [ ] Hungry
- [ ] Tired
- [ ] Bored
- [ ] Emotional

Hunger/Fullness scale:

Ravenous ●●●●●● Stuffed

Protein ○ Carbs ○ Sugar ○
Fat ○ Calories ○ Sodium ○

Snack 3

I ate because I felt:

- [ ] Hungry
- [ ] Tired
- [ ] Bored
- [ ] Emotional

Hunger/Fullness scale:

Ravenous ●●●●●● Stuffed

Protein ○ Carbs ○ Sugar ○
Fat ○ Calories ○ Sodium ○

Vitamins: Yes! [ ]   I forgot... [ ]

Daily Planner

Daily tasks:

♡ ....
♡ ....
♡ ....
♡ ....
♡ ....

My mood:

☹ ☹ 😐 🙂 😄

Hours of sleep:

2	3	4	5	6	7	8	9	10	11	12
☐	☐	☐	☐	☐	☐	☐	☐	☐	☐	☐

Today's affirmation:

....
....

Notes:

Daily schedule:

8.00	
9.00	
10.00	
11.00	
12.00	
1.00	
2.00	
3.00	
4.00	
5.00	
6.00	
7.00	
8.00	
9.00	
10.00	

Food Diary

Breakfast

I ate because I felt:
- [ ] Hungry
- [ ] Bored
- [ ] Tired
- [ ] Emotional

Hunger/Fullness scale:

Ravenous ●●●●●○ Stuffed

Protein · Carbs · Sugar

Fat · Calories · Sodium

Lunch

I ate because I felt:
- [ ] Hungry
- [ ] Bored
- [ ] Tired
- [ ] Emotional

Hunger/Fullness scale:

Ravenous ●●●●●○ Stuffed

Protein · Carbs · Sugar

Fat · Calories · Sodium

Dinner

I ate because I felt:
- [ ] Hungry
- [ ] Bored
- [ ] Tired
- [ ] Emotional

Hunger/Fullness scale:

Ravenous ●●●●●○ Stuffed

Protein · Carbs · Sugar

Fat · Calories · Sodium

Snack 1

I ate because I felt:
- [ ] Hungry
- [ ] Bored
- [ ] Tired
- [ ] Emotional

Hunger/Fullness scale:

Ravenous ●●●●●○ Stuffed

Protein · Carbs · Sugar

Fat · Calories · Sodium

Snack 2

I ate because I felt:
- [ ] Hungry
- [ ] Bored
- [ ] Tired
- [ ] Emotional

Hunger/Fullness scale:

Ravenous ●●●●●○ Stuffed

Protein · Carbs · Sugar

Fat · Calories · Sodium

Snack 3

I ate because I felt:
- [ ] Hungry
- [ ] Bored
- [ ] Tired
- [ ] Emotional

Hunger/Fullness scale:

Ravenous ●●●●●○ Stuffed

Protein · Carbs · Sugar

Fat · Calories · Sodium

Vitamins: Yes! [ ]   I forgot... [ ]

66

Daily Planner

Daily tasks:

♡ ....
♡ ....
♡ ....
♡ ....
♡ ....

My mood:

☹ ☹ 😐 🙂 😃

Hours of sleep:

2 3 4 5 6 7 8 9 10 11 12
☐ ☐ ☐ ☐ ☐ ☐ ☐ ☐ ☐ ☐ ☐

Today's affirmation:

....

....

Notes:

Daily schedule:

8.00	
9.00	
10.00	
11.00	
12.00	
1.00	
2.00	
3.00	
4.00	
5.00	
6.00	
7.00	
8.00	
9.00	
10.00	

Food Diary

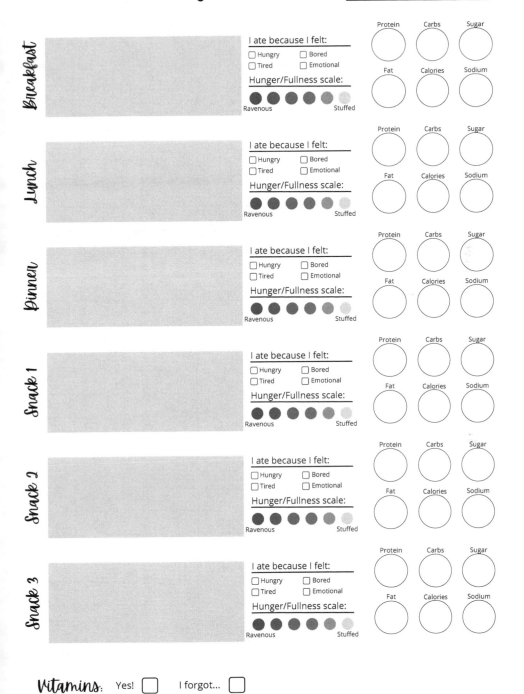

Breakfast

I ate because I felt:
- [ ] Hungry
- [ ] Bored
- [ ] Tired
- [ ] Emotional

Hunger/Fullness scale:

Ravenous — Stuffed

Protein | Carbs | Sugar
Fat | Calories | Sodium

Lunch

I ate because I felt:
- [ ] Hungry
- [ ] Bored
- [ ] Tired
- [ ] Emotional

Hunger/Fullness scale:

Ravenous — Stuffed

Protein | Carbs | Sugar
Fat | Calories | Sodium

Dinner

I ate because I felt:
- [ ] Hungry
- [ ] Bored
- [ ] Tired
- [ ] Emotional

Hunger/Fullness scale:

Ravenous — Stuffed

Protein | Carbs | Sugar
Fat | Calories | Sodium

Snack 1

I ate because I felt:
- [ ] Hungry
- [ ] Bored
- [ ] Tired
- [ ] Emotional

Hunger/Fullness scale:

Ravenous — Stuffed

Protein | Carbs | Sugar
Fat | Calories | Sodium

Snack 2

I ate because I felt:
- [ ] Hungry
- [ ] Bored
- [ ] Tired
- [ ] Emotional

Hunger/Fullness scale:

Ravenous — Stuffed

Protein | Carbs | Sugar
Fat | Calories | Sodium

Snack 3

I ate because I felt:
- [ ] Hungry
- [ ] Bored
- [ ] Tired
- [ ] Emotional

Hunger/Fullness scale:

Ravenous — Stuffed

Protein | Carbs | Sugar
Fat | Calories | Sodium

Vitamins: Yes! [ ] I forgot... [ ]

Daily Planner

Daily tasks:

♡ ....
♡ ....
♡ ....
♡ ....
♡ ....

My mood:

☹ ☹ 😐 ☺ 😃

Hours of sleep:

2	3	4	5	6	7	8	9	10	11	12
☐	☐	☐	☐	☐	☐	☐	☐	☐	☐	☐

Today's affirmation:

....
....

Notes:

Daily schedule:

8.00	
9.00	
10.00	
11.00	
12.00	
1.00	
2.00	
3.00	
4.00	
5.00	
6.00	
7.00	
8.00	
9.00	
10.00	

69

Food Diary

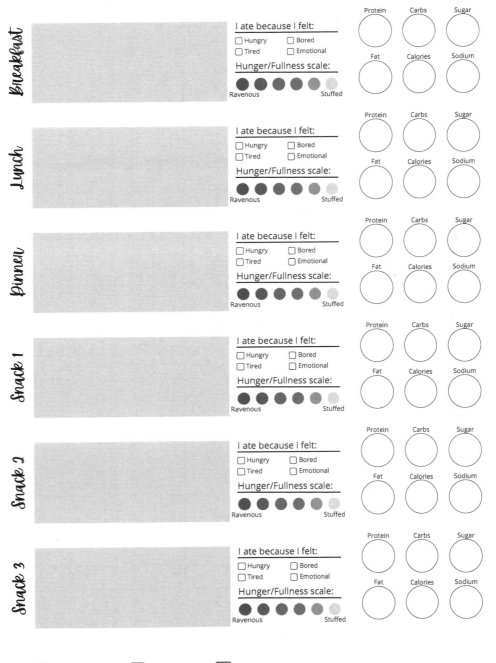

Breakfast

I ate because I felt:
- ☐ Hungry
- ☐ Tired
- ☐ Bored
- ☐ Emotional

Hunger/Fullness scale:

Ravenous ●●●●● Stuffed

Protein · Carbs · Sugar
Fat · Calories · Sodium

Lunch

I ate because I felt:
- ☐ Hungry
- ☐ Tired
- ☐ Bored
- ☐ Emotional

Hunger/Fullness scale:

Ravenous ●●●●● Stuffed

Protein · Carbs · Sugar
Fat · Calories · Sodium

Dinner

I ate because I felt:
- ☐ Hungry
- ☐ Tired
- ☐ Bored
- ☐ Emotional

Hunger/Fullness scale:

Ravenous ●●●●● Stuffed

Protein · Carbs · Sugar
Fat · Calories · Sodium

Snack 1

I ate because I felt:
- ☐ Hungry
- ☐ Tired
- ☐ Bored
- ☐ Emotional

Hunger/Fullness scale:

Ravenous ●●●●● Stuffed

Protein · Carbs · Sugar
Fat · Calories · Sodium

Snack 2

I ate because I felt:
- ☐ Hungry
- ☐ Tired
- ☐ Bored
- ☐ Emotional

Hunger/Fullness scale:

Ravenous ●●●●● Stuffed

Protein · Carbs · Sugar
Fat · Calories · Sodium

Snack 3

I ate because I felt:
- ☐ Hungry
- ☐ Tired
- ☐ Bored
- ☐ Emotional

Hunger/Fullness scale:

Ravenous ●●●●● Stuffed

Protein · Carbs · Sugar
Fat · Calories · Sodium

Vitamins: Yes! ☐   I forgot... ☐

Daily Planner

Daily tasks:

♡ ....
♡ ....
♡ ....
♡ ....
♡ ....

My mood:

☹ ☹ 😐 🙂 😃

Hours of sleep:

2	3	4	5	6	7	8	9	10	11	12
☐	☐	☐	☐	☐	☐	☐	☐	☐	☐	☐

Today's affirmation:

....

....

Notes:

Daily schedule:

8.00	
9.00	
10.00	
11.00	
12.00	
1.00	
2.00	
3.00	
4.00	
5.00	
6.00	
7.00	
8.00	
9.00	
10.00	

Food Diary

Breakfast

I ate because I felt:
- [ ] Hungry
- [ ] Tired
- [ ] Bored
- [ ] Emotional

Hunger/Fullness scale:

Ravenous ●●●●●● Stuffed

Protein Carbs Sugar

Fat Calories Sodium

Lunch

I ate because I felt:
- [ ] Hungry
- [ ] Tired
- [ ] Bored
- [ ] Emotional

Hunger/Fullness scale:

Ravenous ●●●●●● Stuffed

Protein Carbs Sugar

Fat Calories Sodium

Dinner

I ate because I felt:
- [ ] Hungry
- [ ] Tired
- [ ] Bored
- [ ] Emotional

Hunger/Fullness scale:

Ravenous ●●●●●● Stuffed

Protein Carbs Sugar

Fat Calories Sodium

Snack 1

I ate because I felt:
- [ ] Hungry
- [ ] Tired
- [ ] Bored
- [ ] Emotional

Hunger/Fullness scale:

Ravenous ●●●●●● Stuffed

Protein Carbs Sugar

Fat Calories Sodium

Snack 2

I ate because I felt:
- [ ] Hungry
- [ ] Tired
- [ ] Bored
- [ ] Emotional

Hunger/Fullness scale:

Ravenous ●●●●●● Stuffed

Protein Carbs Sugar

Fat Calories Sodium

Snack 3

I ate because I felt:
- [ ] Hungry
- [ ] Tired
- [ ] Bored
- [ ] Emotional

Hunger/Fullness scale:

Ravenous ●●●●●● Stuffed

Protein Carbs Sugar

Fat Calories Sodium

Vitamins: Yes! [ ]   I forgot... [ ]

Daily Planner

Daily tasks:

♡ ....
♡ ....
♡ ....
♡ ....
♡ ....

My mood:

☹ ☹ 😐 🙂 😃

Hours of sleep:

2	3	4	5	6	7	8	9	10	11	12
☐	☐	☐	☐	☐	☐	☐	☐	☐	☐	☐

Today's affirmation:

....

....

Notes:

Daily schedule:

8.00	
9.00	
10.00	
11.00	
12.00	
1.00	
2.00	
3.00	
4.00	
5.00	
6.00	
7.00	
8.00	
9.00	
10.00	

73

Food Diary

Saturday _____

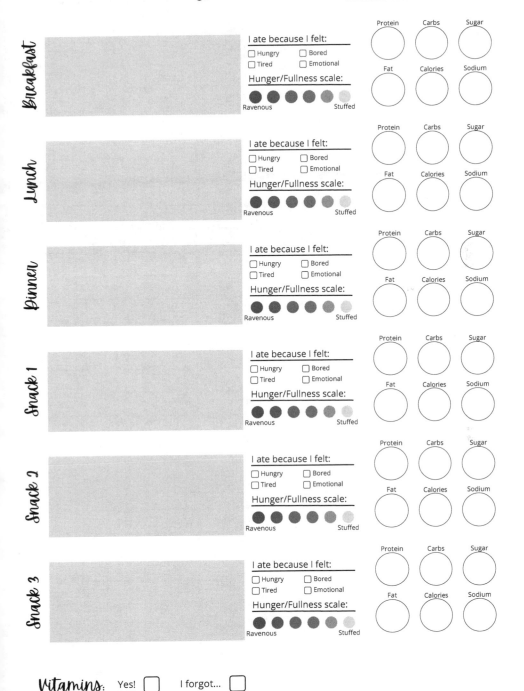

Breakfast

I ate because I felt:
- ☐ Hungry
- ☐ Bored
- ☐ Tired
- ☐ Emotional

Hunger/Fullness scale:

Ravenous ●●●●●○ Stuffed

Protein ○ Carbs ○ Sugar ○
Fat ○ Calories ○ Sodium ○

Lunch

I ate because I felt:
- ☐ Hungry
- ☐ Bored
- ☐ Tired
- ☐ Emotional

Hunger/Fullness scale:

Ravenous ●●●●●○ Stuffed

Protein ○ Carbs ○ Sugar ○
Fat ○ Calories ○ Sodium ○

Dinner

I ate because I felt:
- ☐ Hungry
- ☐ Bored
- ☐ Tired
- ☐ Emotional

Hunger/Fullness scale:

Ravenous ●●●●●○ Stuffed

Protein ○ Carbs ○ Sugar ○
Fat ○ Calories ○ Sodium ○

Snack 1

I ate because I felt:
- ☐ Hungry
- ☐ Bored
- ☐ Tired
- ☐ Emotional

Hunger/Fullness scale:

Ravenous ●●●●●○ Stuffed

Protein ○ Carbs ○ Sugar ○
Fat ○ Calories ○ Sodium ○

Snack 2

I ate because I felt:
- ☐ Hungry
- ☐ Bored
- ☐ Tired
- ☐ Emotional

Hunger/Fullness scale:

Ravenous ●●●●●○ Stuffed

Protein ○ Carbs ○ Sugar ○
Fat ○ Calories ○ Sodium ○

Snack 3

I ate because I felt:
- ☐ Hungry
- ☐ Bored
- ☐ Tired
- ☐ Emotional

Hunger/Fullness scale:

Ravenous ●●●●●○ Stuffed

Protein ○ Carbs ○ Sugar ○
Fat ○ Calories ○ Sodium ○

Vitamins: Yes! ☐   I forgot... ☐

74

Daily Planner

Daily tasks:

♡ ....
♡ ....
♡ ....
♡ ....
♡ ....

My mood:

☹ ☹ 😐 ☺ 😃

Hours of sleep:

2 3 4 5 6 7 8 9 10 11 12
☐ ☐ ☐ ☐ ☐ ☐ ☐ ☐ ☐ ☐ ☐

Today's affirmation:

....

....

Notes:

Daily schedule:

8.00	
9.00	
10.00	
11.00	
12.00	
1.00	
2.00	
3.00	
4.00	
5.00	
6.00	
7.00	
8.00	
9.00	
10.00	

Food Diary

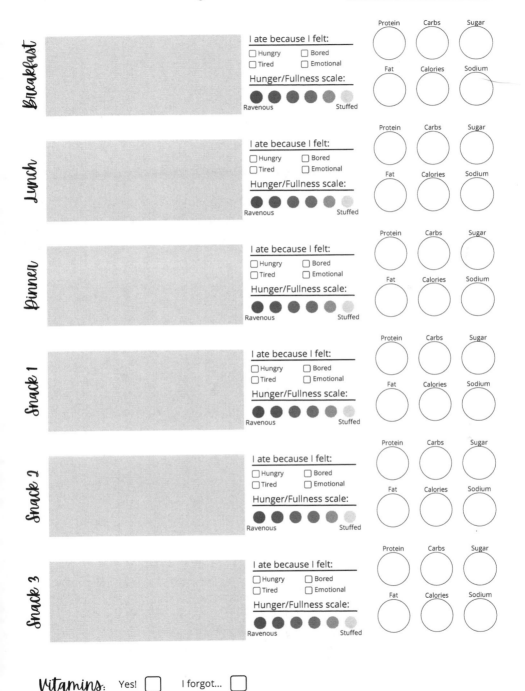

Breakfast

I ate because I felt:
- [ ] Hungry
- [ ] Tired
- [ ] Bored
- [ ] Emotional

Hunger/Fullness scale:

Ravenous ● ● ● ● ● ● Stuffed

Protein | Carbs | Sugar
Fat | Calories | Sodium

Lunch

I ate because I felt:
- [ ] Hungry
- [ ] Tired
- [ ] Bored
- [ ] Emotional

Hunger/Fullness scale:

Ravenous ● ● ● ● ● ● Stuffed

Protein | Carbs | Sugar
Fat | Calories | Sodium

Dinner

I ate because I felt:
- [ ] Hungry
- [ ] Tired
- [ ] Bored
- [ ] Emotional

Hunger/Fullness scale:

Ravenous ● ● ● ● ● ● Stuffed

Protein | Carbs | Sugar
Fat | Calories | Sodium

Snack 1

I ate because I felt:
- [ ] Hungry
- [ ] Tired
- [ ] Bored
- [ ] Emotional

Hunger/Fullness scale:

Ravenous ● ● ● ● ● ● Stuffed

Protein | Carbs | Sugar
Fat | Calories | Sodium

Snack 2

I ate because I felt:
- [ ] Hungry
- [ ] Tired
- [ ] Bored
- [ ] Emotional

Hunger/Fullness scale:

Ravenous ● ● ● ● ● ● Stuffed

Protein | Carbs | Sugar
Fat | Calories | Sodium

Snack 3

I ate because I felt:
- [ ] Hungry
- [ ] Tired
- [ ] Bored
- [ ] Emotional

Hunger/Fullness scale:

Ravenous ● ● ● ● ● ● Stuffed

Protein | Carbs | Sugar
Fat | Calories | Sodium

Vitamins: Yes! [ ]   I forgot... [ ]

Hydration Tracker Week 3

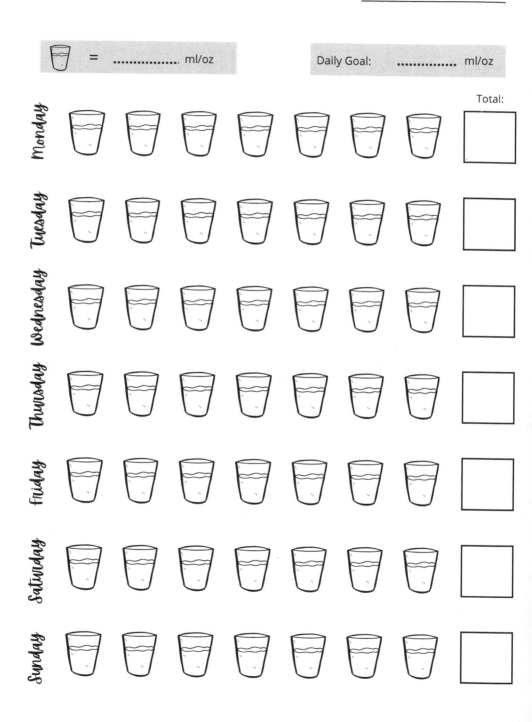

Meal Planner

Week 3

Meals:

Grocery List:

Monday	
Tuesday	
Wednesday	
Thursday	
Friday	
Saturday	
Sunday	

♡ ....
♡ ....
♡ ....
♡ ....
♡ ....
♡ ....
♡ ....
♡ ....
♡ ....
♡ ....
♡ ....
♡ ....
♡ ....
♡ ....
♡ ....
♡ ....
♡ ....
♡ ....
♡ ....
♡ ....
♡ ....

Activity Tracker

Week 3

Daily Target: .... minutes

Minutes:

Monday

....

....

Tuesday

....

....

Wednesday

....

....

Thursday

....

....

Friday

....

....

Saturday

....

....

Sunday

....

....

Habit Tracker

Habit	MON	TUE	WED	THU	FRI	SAT	SUN
	○	○	○	○	○	○	○
	○	○	○	○	○	○	○
	○	○	○	○	○	○	○
	○	○	○	○	○	○	○
	○	○	○	○	○	○	○
	○	○	○	○	○	○	○
	○	○	○	○	○	○	○
	○	○	○	○	○	○	○
	○	○	○	○	○	○	○
	○	○	○	○	○	○	○
	○	○	○	○	○	○	○
	○	○	○	○	○	○	○
	○	○	○	○	○	○	○
	○	○	○	○	○	○	○
	○	○	○	○	○	○	○
	○	○	○	○	○	○	○
	○	○	○	○	○	○	○
	○	○	○	○	○	○	○

Notes:

Your weight is
not your worth.

Weigh-In

Highest Weight

Weight Last Week

Weekly Weight Loss +/-

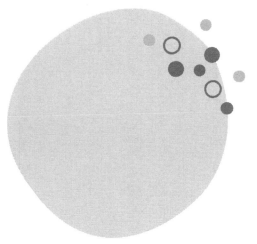

Current Weight

Notes: _____

....

....

Measurements

	Highest	Last Week	This Week	Lost
Neck				
Shoulders				
Chest				
Right Arm				
Left Arm				
Waist				
Hips				
Right Thigh				
Left Thigh				
Right Calf				
Left Calf				

Notes:

....

....

....

Progress Picture

Worthy Then

Worthy Now

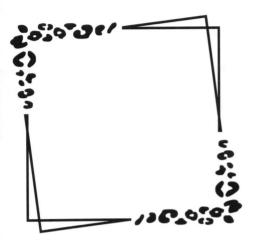
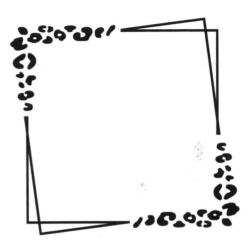

Date: ....

Weight: ....

Date: ....

Weight: ....

Describe how you felt in both pictures:

....

....

....

....

Reflection

Skills I have worked on this week:

....

....

....

....

I still need to be more mindful of:

....

....

....

....

I am thankful for:

....

....

....

....

Next week I will focus more on:

....

....

....

Brain Dump

What's on your mind?

....

....

....

....

....

....

....

....

....

....

....

....

....

....

....

....

....

....

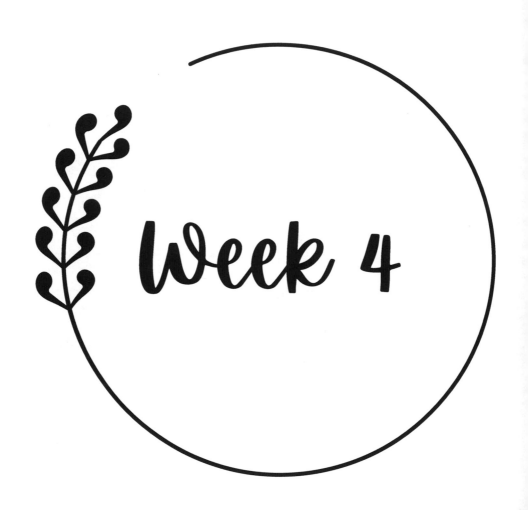

Week 4

Weekly Planner

Priorities:

- ♡ ....
- ♡ ....
- ♡ ....
- ♡ ....
- ♡ ....

To do:

- ☐ ....
- ☐ ....
- ☐ ....
- ☐ ....
- ☐ ....
- ☐ ....
- ☐ ....
- ☐ ....
- ☐ ....
- ☐ ....
- ☐ ....

Notes:

Monday

Tuesday

Wednesday

Thursday

Friday

Saturday

Sunday

Daily Planner

Daily tasks:

♡ ....
♡ ....
♡ ....
♡ ....
♡ ....

My mood:

☹ ☹ 😐 🙂 😀

Hours of sleep:

2	3	4	5	6	7	8	9	10	11	12
☐	☐	☐	☐	☐	☐	☐	☐	☐	☐	☐

Today's affirmation:

....

....

Notes:

Daily schedule:

Time	
8:00	
9:00	
10:00	
11:00	
12:00	
1:00	
2:00	
3:00	
4:00	
5:00	
6:00	
7:00	
8:00	
9:00	
10:00	

89

Food Diary

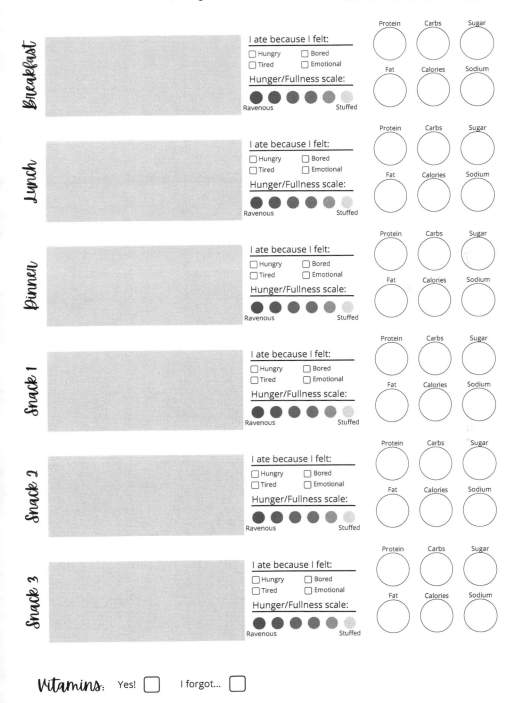

Breakfast

I ate because I felt:
- ☐ Hungry
- ☐ Bored
- ☐ Tired
- ☐ Emotional

Hunger/Fullness scale:
Ravenous ●●●●●○ Stuffed

Protein Carbs Sugar
Fat Calories Sodium

Lunch

I ate because I felt:
- ☐ Hungry
- ☐ Bored
- ☐ Tired
- ☐ Emotional

Hunger/Fullness scale:
Ravenous ●●●●●○ Stuffed

Protein Carbs Sugar
Fat Calories Sodium

Dinner

I ate because I felt:
- ☐ Hungry
- ☐ Bored
- ☐ Tired
- ☐ Emotional

Hunger/Fullness scale:
Ravenous ●●●●●○ Stuffed

Protein Carbs Sugar
Fat Calories Sodium

Snack 1

I ate because I felt:
- ☐ Hungry
- ☐ Bored
- ☐ Tired
- ☐ Emotional

Hunger/Fullness scale:
Ravenous ●●●●●○ Stuffed

Protein Carbs Sugar
Fat Calories Sodium

Snack 2

I ate because I felt:
- ☐ Hungry
- ☐ Bored
- ☐ Tired
- ☐ Emotional

Hunger/Fullness scale:
Ravenous ●●●●●○ Stuffed

Protein Carbs Sugar
Fat Calories Sodium

Snack 3

I ate because I felt:
- ☐ Hungry
- ☐ Bored
- ☐ Tired
- ☐ Emotional

Hunger/Fullness scale:
Ravenous ●●●●●○ Stuffed

Protein Carbs Sugar
Fat Calories Sodium

Vitamins: Yes! ☐   I forgot... ☐

Daily Planner

Daily tasks:

♡ ....
♡ ....
♡ ....
♡ ....
♡ ....

My mood:

☹ ☹ 😐 🙂 😃

Hours of sleep:

2 3 4 5 6 7 8 9 10 11 12
☐ ☐ ☐ ☐ ☐ ☐ ☐ ☐ ☐ ☐ ☐

Today's affirmation:

....
....

Notes:

Daily schedule:

8:00	
9:00	
10:00	
11:00	
12:00	
1:00	
2:00	
3:00	
4:00	
5:00	
6:00	
7:00	
8:00	
9:00	
10:00	

91

Food Diary

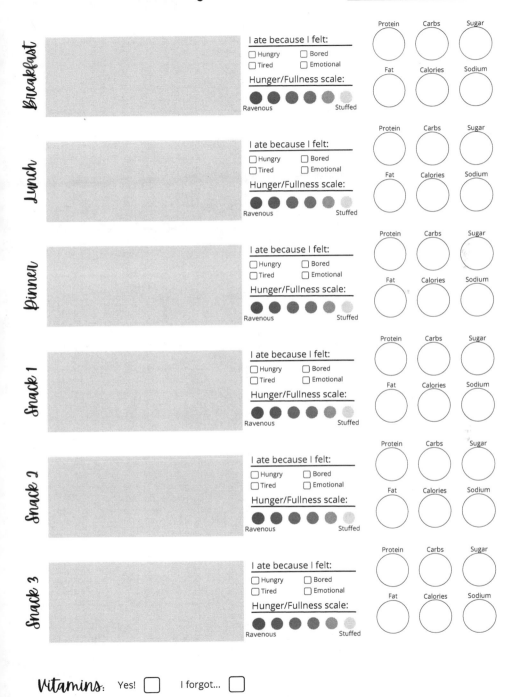

Breakfast

I ate because I felt:
- ☐ Hungry
- ☐ Tired
- ☐ Bored
- ☐ Emotional

Hunger/Fullness scale:

Ravenous ●●●●● Stuffed

Protein ◯ Carbs ◯ Sugar ◯
Fat ◯ Calories ◯ Sodium ◯

Lunch

I ate because I felt:
- ☐ Hungry
- ☐ Tired
- ☐ Bored
- ☐ Emotional

Hunger/Fullness scale:

Ravenous ●●●●● Stuffed

Protein ◯ Carbs ◯ Sugar ◯
Fat ◯ Calories ◯ Sodium ◯

Dinner

I ate because I felt:
- ☐ Hungry
- ☐ Tired
- ☐ Bored
- ☐ Emotional

Hunger/Fullness scale:

Ravenous ●●●●● Stuffed

Protein ◯ Carbs ◯ Sugar ◯
Fat ◯ Calories ◯ Sodium ◯

Snack 1

I ate because I felt:
- ☐ Hungry
- ☐ Tired
- ☐ Bored
- ☐ Emotional

Hunger/Fullness scale:

Ravenous ●●●●● Stuffed

Protein ◯ Carbs ◯ Sugar ◯
Fat ◯ Calories ◯ Sodium ◯

Snack 2

I ate because I felt:
- ☐ Hungry
- ☐ Tired
- ☐ Bored
- ☐ Emotional

Hunger/Fullness scale:

Ravenous ●●●●● Stuffed

Protein ◯ Carbs ◯ Sugar ◯
Fat ◯ Calories ◯ Sodium ◯

Snack 3

I ate because I felt:
- ☐ Hungry
- ☐ Tired
- ☐ Bored
- ☐ Emotional

Hunger/Fullness scale:

Ravenous ●●●●● Stuffed

Protein ◯ Carbs ◯ Sugar ◯
Fat ◯ Calories ◯ Sodium ◯

Vitamins: Yes! ☐   I forgot... ☐

Daily Planner

Daily tasks:

♡ ....
♡ ....
♡ ....
♡ ....
♡ ....

My mood:

😢 😟 😐 🙂 😄

Hours of sleep:

2   3   4   5   6   7   8   9   10   11   12
☐ ☐ ☐ ☐ ☐ ☐ ☐ ☐ ☐ ☐ ☐

Today's affirmation:

....

....

Notes:

Daily schedule:

Time	
8.00	
9.00	
10.00	
11.00	
12.00	
1.00	
2.00	
3.00	
4.00	
5.00	
6.00	
7.00	
8.00	
9.00	
10.00	

Food Diary

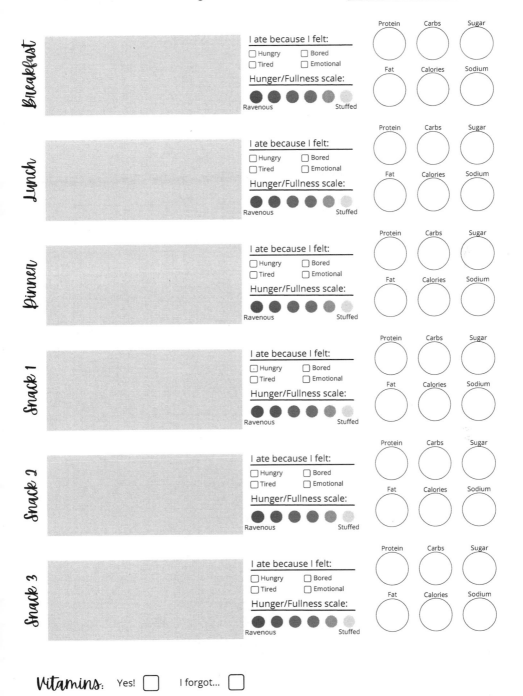

Breakfast

I ate because I felt:
- [ ] Hungry
- [ ] Tired
- [ ] Bored
- [ ] Emotional

Hunger/Fullness scale:

Ravenous   Stuffed

Protein   Carbs   Sugar

Fat   Calories   Sodium

Lunch

I ate because I felt:
- [ ] Hungry
- [ ] Tired
- [ ] Bored
- [ ] Emotional

Hunger/Fullness scale:

Ravenous   Stuffed

Protein   Carbs   Sugar

Fat   Calories   Sodium

Dinner

I ate because I felt:
- [ ] Hungry
- [ ] Tired
- [ ] Bored
- [ ] Emotional

Hunger/Fullness scale:

Ravenous   Stuffed

Protein   Carbs   Sugar

Fat   Calories   Sodium

Snack 1

I ate because I felt:
- [ ] Hungry
- [ ] Tired
- [ ] Bored
- [ ] Emotional

Hunger/Fullness scale:

Ravenous   Stuffed

Protein   Carbs   Sugar

Fat   Calories   Sodium

Snack 2

I ate because I felt:
- [ ] Hungry
- [ ] Tired
- [ ] Bored
- [ ] Emotional

Hunger/Fullness scale:

Ravenous   Stuffed

Protein   Carbs   Sugar

Fat   Calories   Sodium

Snack 3

I ate because I felt:
- [ ] Hungry
- [ ] Tired
- [ ] Bored
- [ ] Emotional

Hunger/Fullness scale:

Ravenous   Stuffed

Protein   Carbs   Sugar

Fat   Calories   Sodium

Vitamins: Yes! [ ]   I forgot... [ ]

Daily Planner

Daily tasks:

♡ ....
♡ ....
♡ ....
♡ ....
♡ ....

My mood:

☹ ☹ 😐 🙂 😃

Hours of sleep:

2 3 4 5 6 7 8 9 10 11 12
☐ ☐ ☐ ☐ ☐ ☐ ☐ ☐ ☐ ☐ ☐

Today's affirmation:

....

....

Notes:

Daily schedule:

8.00	
9.00	
10.00	
11.00	
12.00	
1.00	
2.00	
3.00	
4.00	
5.00	
6.00	
7.00	
8.00	
9.00	
10.00	

Food Diary

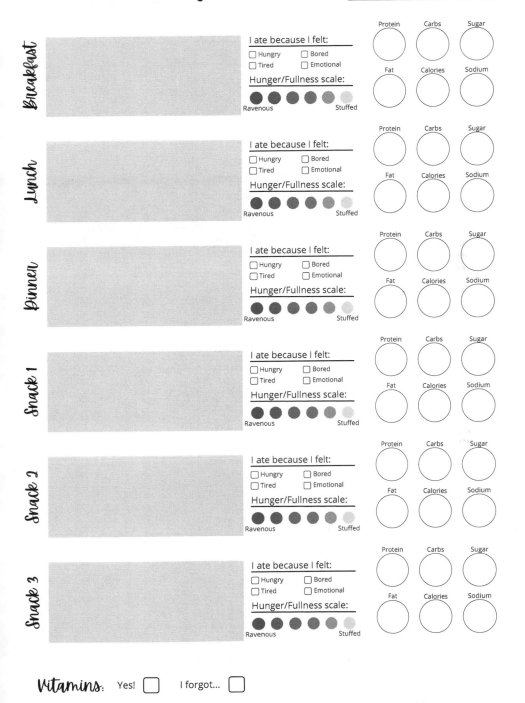

Breakfast

I ate because I felt:
- [ ] Hungry
- [ ] Tired
- [ ] Bored
- [ ] Emotional

Hunger/Fullness scale:

Ravenous · Stuffed

Protein · Carbs · Sugar
Fat · Calories · Sodium

Lunch

I ate because I felt:
- [ ] Hungry
- [ ] Tired
- [ ] Bored
- [ ] Emotional

Hunger/Fullness scale:

Ravenous · Stuffed

Protein · Carbs · Sugar
Fat · Calories · Sodium

Dinner

I ate because I felt:
- [ ] Hungry
- [ ] Tired
- [ ] Bored
- [ ] Emotional

Hunger/Fullness scale:

Ravenous · Stuffed

Protein · Carbs · Sugar
Fat · Calories · Sodium

Snack 1

I ate because I felt:
- [ ] Hungry
- [ ] Tired
- [ ] Bored
- [ ] Emotional

Hunger/Fullness scale:

Ravenous · Stuffed

Protein · Carbs · Sugar
Fat · Calories · Sodium

Snack 2

I ate because I felt:
- [ ] Hungry
- [ ] Tired
- [ ] Bored
- [ ] Emotional

Hunger/Fullness scale:

Ravenous · Stuffed

Protein · Carbs · Sugar
Fat · Calories · Sodium

Snack 3

I ate because I felt:
- [ ] Hungry
- [ ] Tired
- [ ] Bored
- [ ] Emotional

Hunger/Fullness scale:

Ravenous · Stuffed

Protein · Carbs · Sugar
Fat · Calories · Sodium

Vitamins: Yes! [ ]   I forgot... [ ]

Daily Planner

Friday

Daily tasks:

♡ ....
♡ ....
♡ ....
♡ ....
♡ ....

My mood:

😢 😟 😐 🙂 😄

Hours of sleep:

2	3	4	5	6	7	8	9	10	11	12
☐	☐	☐	☐	☐	☐	☐	☐	☐	☐	☐

Today's affirmation:

....
....

Notes:

Daily schedule:

8.00	
9.00	
10.00	
11.00	
12.00	
1.00	
2.00	
3.00	
4.00	
5.00	
6.00	
7.00	
8.00	
9.00	
10.00	

97

Food Diary

Breakfast

I ate because I felt:
- [ ] Hungry
- [ ] Tired
- [ ] Bored
- [ ] Emotional

Hunger/Fullness scale:

Ravenous ●●●●●○ Stuffed

Protein | Carbs | Sugar

Fat | Calories | Sodium

Lunch

I ate because I felt:
- [ ] Hungry
- [ ] Tired
- [ ] Bored
- [ ] Emotional

Hunger/Fullness scale:

Ravenous ●●●●●○ Stuffed

Protein | Carbs | Sugar

Fat | Calories | Sodium

Dinner

I ate because I felt:
- [ ] Hungry
- [ ] Tired
- [ ] Bored
- [ ] Emotional

Hunger/Fullness scale:

Ravenous ●●●●●○ Stuffed

Protein | Carbs | Sugar

Fat | Calories | Sodium

Snack 1

I ate because I felt:
- [ ] Hungry
- [ ] Tired
- [ ] Bored
- [ ] Emotional

Hunger/Fullness scale:

Ravenous ●●●●●○ Stuffed

Protein | Carbs | Sugar

Fat | Calories | Sodium

Snack 2

I ate because I felt:
- [ ] Hungry
- [ ] Tired
- [ ] Bored
- [ ] Emotional

Hunger/Fullness scale:

Ravenous ●●●●●○ Stuffed

Protein | Carbs | Sugar

Fat | Calories | Sodium

Snack 3

I ate because I felt:
- [ ] Hungry
- [ ] Tired
- [ ] Bored
- [ ] Emotional

Hunger/Fullness scale:

Ravenous ●●●●●○ Stuffed

Protein | Carbs | Sugar

Fat | Calories | Sodium

Vitamins: Yes! [ ]   I forgot... [ ]

Daily Planner

Daily tasks:

♡ ....
♡ ....
♡ ....
♡ ....
♡ ....

My mood:

☹ ☹ 😐 🙂 😃

Hours of sleep:

| 2 | 3 | 4 | 5 | 6 | 7 | 8 | 9 | 10 | 11 | 12 |
| ☐ | ☐ | ☐ | ☐ | ☐ | ☐ | ☐ | ☐ | ☐ | ☐ | ☐ |

Today's affirmation:

....
....

Notes:

Daily schedule:

8.00	
9.00	
10.00	
11.00	
12.00	
1.00	
2.00	
3.00	
4.00	
5.00	
6.00	
7.00	
8.00	
9.00	
10.00	

Food Diary

Breakfast

I ate because I felt:
- [ ] Hungry
- [ ] Tired
- [ ] Bored
- [ ] Emotional

Hunger/Fullness scale:

Ravenous ●●●●●○ Stuffed

Protein

Carbs

Sugar

Fat

Calories

Sodium

Lunch

I ate because I felt:
- [ ] Hungry
- [ ] Tired
- [ ] Bored
- [ ] Emotional

Hunger/Fullness scale:

Ravenous ●●●●●○ Stuffed

Protein

Carbs

Sugar

Fat

Calories

Sodium

Dinner

I ate because I felt:
- [ ] Hungry
- [ ] Tired
- [ ] Bored
- [ ] Emotional

Hunger/Fullness scale:

Ravenous ●●●●●○ Stuffed

Protein

Carbs

Sugar

Fat

Calories

Sodium

Snack 1

I ate because I felt:
- [ ] Hungry
- [ ] Tired
- [ ] Bored
- [ ] Emotional

Hunger/Fullness scale:

Ravenous ●●●●●○ Stuffed

Protein

Carbs

Sugar

Fat

Calories

Sodium

Snack 2

I ate because I felt:
- [ ] Hungry
- [ ] Tired
- [ ] Bored
- [ ] Emotional

Hunger/Fullness scale:

Ravenous ●●●●●○ Stuffed

Protein

Carbs

Sugar

Fat

Calories

Sodium

Snack 3

I ate because I felt:
- [ ] Hungry
- [ ] Tired
- [ ] Bored
- [ ] Emotional

Hunger/Fullness scale:

Ravenous ●●●●●○ Stuffed

Protein

Carbs

Sugar

Fat

Calories

Sodium

Vitamins: Yes! [ ]   I forgot... [ ]

Daily Planner

<u>Sunday</u>

Daily tasks:

♡ ....
♡ ....
♡ ....
♡ ....
♡ ....

My mood:

☹ ☹ 😐 🙂 😀

Hours of sleep:

2	3	4	5	6	7	8	9	10	11	12
☐	☐	☐	☐	☐	☐	☐	☐	☐	☐	☐

Today's affirmation:

....
....

Notes:

Daily schedule:

8.00	
9.00	
10.00	
11.00	
12.00	
1.00	
2.00	
3.00	
4.00	
5.00	
6.00	
7.00	
8.00	
9.00	
10.00	

Food Diary

Breakfast

I ate because I felt:

☐ Hungry   ☐ Bored
☐ Tired   ☐ Emotional

Hunger/Fullness scale:

Ravenous ●●●●● Stuffed

Protein   Carbs   Sugar

Fat   Calories   Sodium

Lunch

I ate because I felt:

☐ Hungry   ☐ Bored
☐ Tired   ☐ Emotional

Hunger/Fullness scale:

Ravenous ●●●●● Stuffed

Protein   Carbs   Sugar

Fat   Calories   Sodium

Dinner

I ate because I felt:

☐ Hungry   ☐ Bored
☐ Tired   ☐ Emotional

Hunger/Fullness scale:

Ravenous ●●●●● Stuffed

Protein   Carbs   Sugar

Fat   Calories   Sodium

Snack 1

I ate because I felt:

☐ Hungry   ☐ Bored
☐ Tired   ☐ Emotional

Hunger/Fullness scale:

Ravenous ●●●●● Stuffed

Protein   Carbs   Sugar

Fat   Calories   Sodium

Snack 2

I ate because I felt:

☐ Hungry   ☐ Bored
☐ Tired   ☐ Emotional

Hunger/Fullness scale:

Ravenous ●●●●● Stuffed

Protein   Carbs   Sugar

Fat   Calories   Sodium

Snack 3

I ate because I felt:

☐ Hungry   ☐ Bored
☐ Tired   ☐ Emotional

Hunger/Fullness scale:

Ravenous ●●●●● Stuffed

Protein   Carbs   Sugar

Fat   Calories   Sodium

Vitamins: Yes! ☐   I forgot... ☐

Hydration Tracker

Week 4

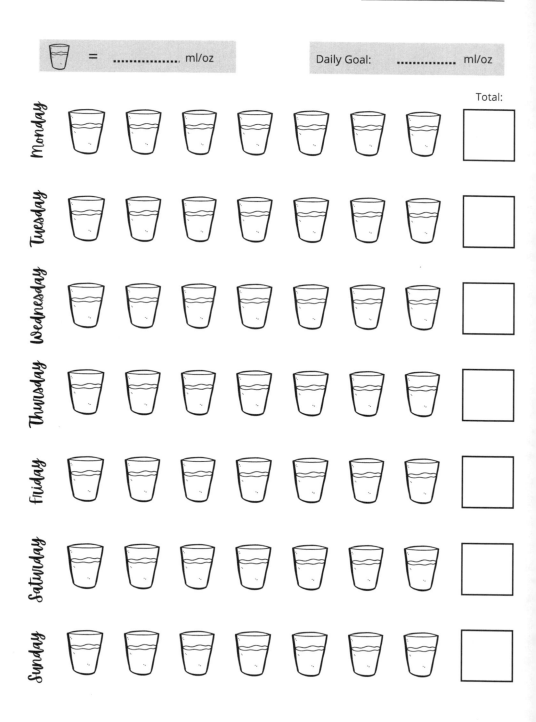

= ...., ml/oz

Daily Goal: .... ml/oz

Monday — Total:

Tuesday

Wednesday

Thursday

Friday

Saturday

Sunday

Meal Planner

Meals:

Grocery List:

Monday

Tuesday

Wednesday

Thursday

Friday

Saturday

Sunday

♡ ....
♡ ....
♡ ....
♡ ....
♡ ....
♡ ....
♡ ....
♡ ....
♡ ....
♡ ....
♡ ....
♡ ....
♡ ....
♡ ....
♡ ....
♡ ....
♡ ....
♡ ....
♡ ....
♡ ....
♡ ....
♡ ....

Activity Tracker

Week 4

Daily Target: .... minutes

Minutes:

Monday

Tuesday

Wednesday

Thursday

Friday

Saturday

Sunday

Habit Tracker

Habit	MON	TUE	WED	THU	FRI	SAT	SUN
	○	○	○	○	○	○	○
	○	○	○	○	○	○	○
	○	○	○	○	○	○	○
	○	○	○	○	○	○	○
	○	○	○	○	○	○	○
	○	○	○	○	○	○	○
	○	○	○	○	○	○	○
	○	○	○	○	○	○	○
	○	○	○	○	○	○	○
	○	○	○	○	○	○	○
	○	○	○	○	○	○	○
	○	○	○	○	○	○	○
	○	○	○	○	○	○	○
	○	○	○	○	○	○	○
	○	○	○	○	○	○	○
	○	○	○	○	○	○	○
	○	○	○	○	○	○	○
	○	○	○	○	○	○	○

Notes:

They might as well call it 'Bariatric Searchery' as you will be looking for new ways to change your life.

Weigh-In

 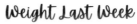

Highest Weight

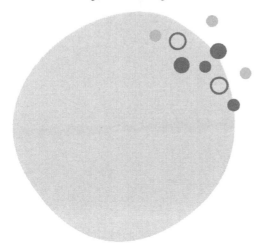

Weight Last Week

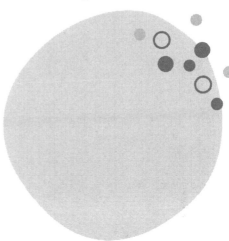

Weekly Weight Loss +/-

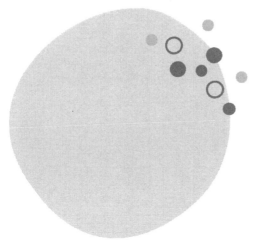

Current Weight

Notes:

....

....

Measurements

	Highest	Last Week	This Week	Lost
Neck				
Shoulders				
Chest				
Right Arm				
Left Arm				
Waist				
Hips				
Right Thigh				
Left Thigh				
Right Calf				
Left Calf				

Notes:

....

....

....

Progress Picture

Worthy Then   Worthy Now

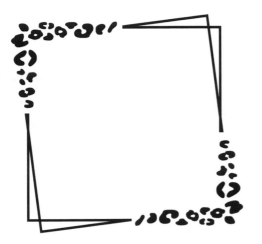 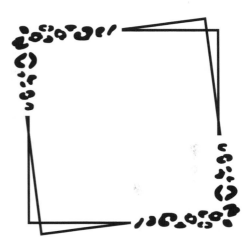

Date: ....   Date: ....

Weight: ....   Weight: ....

Describe how you felt in both pictures: _____

....

....

....

....

Reflection

Skills I have worked on this week:

....

....

....

....

I still need to be more mindful of:

....

....

....

....

I am thankful for:

....

....

....

....

Next week I will focus more on:

....

....

....

Brain Dump

What's on your mind?

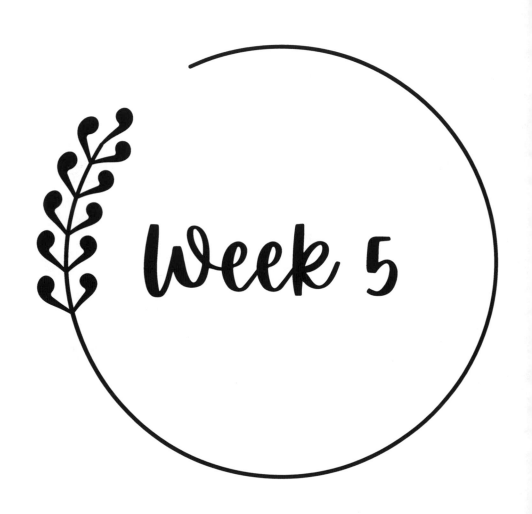

Week 5

Weekly Planner

Priorities:

♡ ....
♡ ....
♡ ....
♡ ....
♡ ....

To do:

☐ ....
☐ ....
☐ ....
☐ ....
☐ ....
☐ ....
☐ ....
☐ ....
☐ ....
☐ ....
☐ ....

Notes:

Monday

Tuesday

Wednesday

Thursday

Friday

Saturday

Sunday

Daily Planner

Daily tasks:

- ♡ ....
- ♡ ....
- ♡ ....
- ♡ ....
- ♡ ....

My mood:

☹ 🙁 😐 🙂 😀

Hours of sleep:

2 3 4 5 6 7 8 9 10 11 12
☐ ☐ ☐ ☐ ☐ ☐ ☐ ☐ ☐ ☐ ☐

Today's affirmation:

....

....

Notes:

Daily schedule:

8.00	
9.00	
10.00	
11.00	
12.00	
1.00	
2.00	
3.00	
4.00	
5.00	
6.00	
7.00	
8.00	
9.00	
10.00	

Food Diary

Breakfast

I ate because I felt:

- ☐ Hungry
- ☐ Tired
- ☐ Bored
- ☐ Emotional

Hunger/Fullness scale:

Ravenous ●●●●●○ Stuffed

Protein · Carbs · Sugar

Fat · Calories · Sodium

Lunch

I ate because I felt:

- ☐ Hungry
- ☐ Tired
- ☐ Bored
- ☐ Emotional

Hunger/Fullness scale:

Ravenous ●●●●●○ Stuffed

Protein · Carbs · Sugar

Fat · Calories · Sodium

Dinner

I ate because I felt:

- ☐ Hungry
- ☐ Tired
- ☐ Bored
- ☐ Emotional

Hunger/Fullness scale:

Ravenous ●●●●●○ Stuffed

Protein · Carbs · Sugar

Fat · Calories · Sodium

Snack 1

I ate because I felt:

- ☐ Hungry
- ☐ Tired
- ☐ Bored
- ☐ Emotional

Hunger/Fullness scale:

Ravenous ●●●●●○ Stuffed

Protein · Carbs · Sugar

Fat · Calories · Sodium

Snack 2

I ate because I felt:

- ☐ Hungry
- ☐ Tired
- ☐ Bored
- ☐ Emotional

Hunger/Fullness scale:

Ravenous ●●●●●○ Stuffed

Protein · Carbs · Sugar

Fat · Calories · Sodium

Snack 3

I ate because I felt:

- ☐ Hungry
- ☐ Tired
- ☐ Bored
- ☐ Emotional

Hunger/Fullness scale:

Ravenous ●●●●●○ Stuffed

Protein · Carbs · Sugar

Fat · Calories · Sodium

Vitamins: Yes! ☐   I forgot... ☐

Daily Planner

Daily tasks:

♡ ....
♡ ....
♡ ....
♡ ....
♡ ....

My mood:

☹ ☹ 😐 🙂 😃

Hours of sleep:

2	3	4	5	6	7	8	9	10	11	12
☐	☐	☐	☐	☐	☐	☐	☐	☐	☐	☐

Today's affirmation:

....

....

Notes:

Daily schedule:

Time	
8.00	
9.00	
10.00	
11.00	
12.00	
1.00	
2.00	
3.00	
4.00	
5.00	
6.00	
7.00	
8.00	
9.00	
10.00	

Food Diary

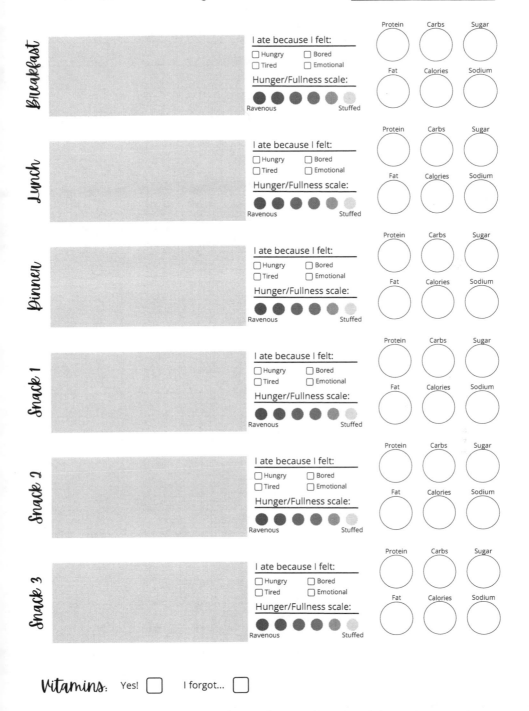

Breakfast

I ate because I felt:
- [ ] Hungry
- [ ] Tired
- [ ] Bored
- [ ] Emotional

Hunger/Fullness scale:
Ravenous ●●●●●○ Stuffed

Protein | Carbs | Sugar
Fat | Calories | Sodium

Lunch

I ate because I felt:
- [ ] Hungry
- [ ] Tired
- [ ] Bored
- [ ] Emotional

Hunger/Fullness scale:
Ravenous ●●●●●○ Stuffed

Protein | Carbs | Sugar
Fat | Calories | Sodium

Dinner

I ate because I felt:
- [ ] Hungry
- [ ] Tired
- [ ] Bored
- [ ] Emotional

Hunger/Fullness scale:
Ravenous ●●●●●○ Stuffed

Protein | Carbs | Sugar
Fat | Calories | Sodium

Snack 1

I ate because I felt:
- [ ] Hungry
- [ ] Tired
- [ ] Bored
- [ ] Emotional

Hunger/Fullness scale:
Ravenous ●●●●●○ Stuffed

Protein | Carbs | Sugar
Fat | Calories | Sodium

Snack 2

I ate because I felt:
- [ ] Hungry
- [ ] Tired
- [ ] Bored
- [ ] Emotional

Hunger/Fullness scale:
Ravenous ●●●●●○ Stuffed

Protein | Carbs | Sugar
Fat | Calories | Sodium

Snack 3

I ate because I felt:
- [ ] Hungry
- [ ] Tired
- [ ] Bored
- [ ] Emotional

Hunger/Fullness scale:
Ravenous ●●●●●○ Stuffed

Protein | Carbs | Sugar
Fat | Calories | Sodium

Vitamins: Yes! [ ]   I forgot... [ ]

Daily Planner

Daily tasks:

♡ ....
♡ ....
♡ ....
♡ ....
♡ ....

My mood:

Hours of sleep:

2 3 4 5 6 7 8 9 10 11 12
☐ ☐ ☐ ☐ ☐ ☐ ☐ ☐ ☐ ☐ ☐

Today's affirmation:

....

....

Notes:

Daily schedule:

8.00	
9.00	
10.00	
11.00	
12.00	
1.00	
2.00	
3.00	
4.00	
5.00	
6.00	
7.00	
8.00	
9.00	
10.00	

119

Food Diary

Breakfast

I ate because I felt:
- [ ] Hungry
- [ ] Tired
- [ ] Bored
- [ ] Emotional

Hunger/Fullness scale:

Ravenous ●●●●●● Stuffed

Protein | Carbs | Sugar
Fat | Calories | Sodium

Lunch

I ate because I felt:
- [ ] Hungry
- [ ] Tired
- [ ] Bored
- [ ] Emotional

Hunger/Fullness scale:

Ravenous ●●●●●● Stuffed

Protein | Carbs | Sugar
Fat | Calories | Sodium

Dinner

I ate because I felt:
- [ ] Hungry
- [ ] Tired
- [ ] Bored
- [ ] Emotional

Hunger/Fullness scale:

Ravenous ●●●●●● Stuffed

Protein | Carbs | Sugar
Fat | Calories | Sodium

Snack 1

I ate because I felt:
- [ ] Hungry
- [ ] Tired
- [ ] Bored
- [ ] Emotional

Hunger/Fullness scale:

Ravenous ●●●●●● Stuffed

Protein | Carbs | Sugar
Fat | Calories | Sodium

Snack 2

I ate because I felt:
- [ ] Hungry
- [ ] Tired
- [ ] Bored
- [ ] Emotional

Hunger/Fullness scale:

Ravenous ●●●●●● Stuffed

Protein | Carbs | Sugar
Fat | Calories | Sodium

Snack 3

I ate because I felt:
- [ ] Hungry
- [ ] Tired
- [ ] Bored
- [ ] Emotional

Hunger/Fullness scale:

Ravenous ●●●●●● Stuffed

Protein | Carbs | Sugar
Fat | Calories | Sodium

Vitamins: Yes! [ ]   I forgot... [ ]

Daily Planner

Daily tasks:

♡ ....

♡ ....

♡ ....

♡ ....

♡ ....

My mood:

☹ ☹ 😐 ☺ 😃

Hours of sleep:

2	3	4	5	6	7	8	9	10	11	12
☐	☐	☐	☐	☐	☐	☐	☐	☐	☐	☐

Today's affirmation:

....

....

Notes:

Daily schedule:

8:00	
9:00	
10:00	
11:00	
12:00	
1:00	
2:00	
3:00	
4:00	
5:00	
6:00	
7:00	
8:00	
9:00	
10:00	

Food Diary

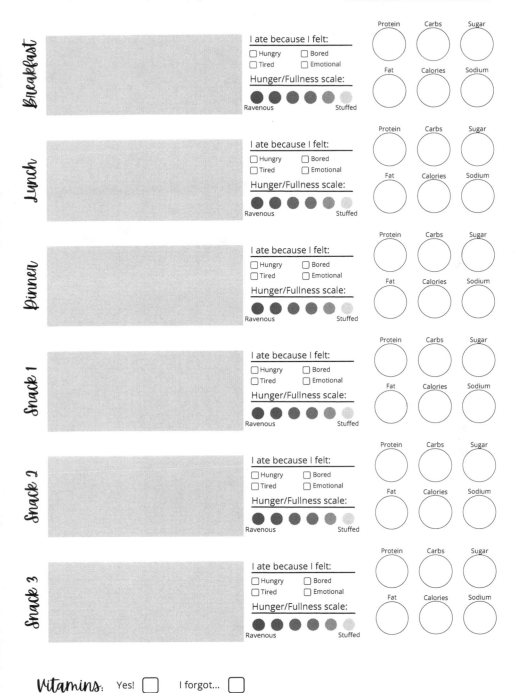

Breakfast

I ate because I felt:
- ☐ Hungry
- ☐ Tired
- ☐ Bored
- ☐ Emotional

Hunger/Fullness scale:
Ravenous ●●●●●○ Stuffed

Protein | Carbs | Sugar
Fat | Calories | Sodium

Lunch

I ate because I felt:
- ☐ Hungry
- ☐ Tired
- ☐ Bored
- ☐ Emotional

Hunger/Fullness scale:
Ravenous ●●●●●○ Stuffed

Protein | Carbs | Sugar
Fat | Calories | Sodium

Dinner

I ate because I felt:
- ☐ Hungry
- ☐ Tired
- ☐ Bored
- ☐ Emotional

Hunger/Fullness scale:
Ravenous ●●●●●○ Stuffed

Protein | Carbs | Sugar
Fat | Calories | Sodium

Snack 1

I ate because I felt:
- ☐ Hungry
- ☐ Tired
- ☐ Bored
- ☐ Emotional

Hunger/Fullness scale:
Ravenous ●●●●●○ Stuffed

Protein | Carbs | Sugar
Fat | Calories | Sodium

Snack 2

I ate because I felt:
- ☐ Hungry
- ☐ Tired
- ☐ Bored
- ☐ Emotional

Hunger/Fullness scale:
Ravenous ●●●●●○ Stuffed

Protein | Carbs | Sugar
Fat | Calories | Sodium

Snack 3

I ate because I felt:
- ☐ Hungry
- ☐ Tired
- ☐ Bored
- ☐ Emotional

Hunger/Fullness scale:
Ravenous ●●●●●○ Stuffed

Protein | Carbs | Sugar
Fat | Calories | Sodium

Vitamins: Yes! ☐ I forgot... ☐

Daily Planner

Friday

Daily tasks:

♡ ....
♡ ....
♡ ....
♡ ....
♡ ....

My mood:

☹ ☹ 😐 🙂 😀

Hours of sleep:

2	3	4	5	6	7	8	9	10	11	12
☐	☐	☐	☐	☐	☐	☐	☐	☐	☐	☐

Today's affirmation:

....

....

Notes:

Daily schedule:

8:00	
9:00	
10:00	
11:00	
12:00	
1:00	
2:00	
3:00	
4:00	
5:00	
6:00	
7:00	
8:00	
9:00	
10:00	

123

Food Diary

Breakfast

I ate because I felt:
- ☐ Hungry ☐ Bored
- ☐ Tired ☐ Emotional

Hunger/Fullness scale:

Ravenous ●●●●●● Stuffed

Protein ○ Carbs ○ Sugar ○
Fat ○ Calories ○ Sodium ○

Lunch

I ate because I felt:
- ☐ Hungry ☐ Bored
- ☐ Tired ☐ Emotional

Hunger/Fullness scale:

Ravenous ●●●●●● Stuffed

Protein ○ Carbs ○ Sugar ○
Fat ○ Calories ○ Sodium ○

Dinner

I ate because I felt:
- ☐ Hungry ☐ Bored
- ☐ Tired ☐ Emotional

Hunger/Fullness scale:

Ravenous ●●●●●● Stuffed

Protein ○ Carbs ○ Sugar ○
Fat ○ Calories ○ Sodium ○

Snack 1

I ate because I felt:
- ☐ Hungry ☐ Bored
- ☐ Tired ☐ Emotional

Hunger/Fullness scale:

Ravenous ●●●●●● Stuffed

Protein ○ Carbs ○ Sugar ○
Fat ○ Calories ○ Sodium ○

Snack 2

I ate because I felt:
- ☐ Hungry ☐ Bored
- ☐ Tired ☐ Emotional

Hunger/Fullness scale:

Ravenous ●●●●●● Stuffed

Protein ○ Carbs ○ Sugar ○
Fat ○ Calories ○ Sodium ○

Snack 3

I ate because I felt:
- ☐ Hungry ☐ Bored
- ☐ Tired ☐ Emotional

Hunger/Fullness scale:

Ravenous ●●●●●● Stuffed

Protein ○ Carbs ○ Sugar ○
Fat ○ Calories ○ Sodium ○

Vitamins: Yes! ☐   I forgot... ☐

124

Daily Planner

Daily tasks:

♡ ....

♡ ....

♡ ....

♡ ....

♡ ....

My mood:

😢 😣 😐 🙂 😄

Hours of sleep:

2	3	4	5	6	7	8	9	10	11	12
☐	☐	☐	☐	☐	☐	☐	☐	☐	☐	☐

Today's affirmation:

....

....

Notes:

Daily schedule:

8.00	
9.00	
10.00	
11.00	
12.00	
1.00	
2.00	
3.00	
4.00	
5.00	
6.00	
7.00	
8.00	
9.00	
10.00	

Food Diary

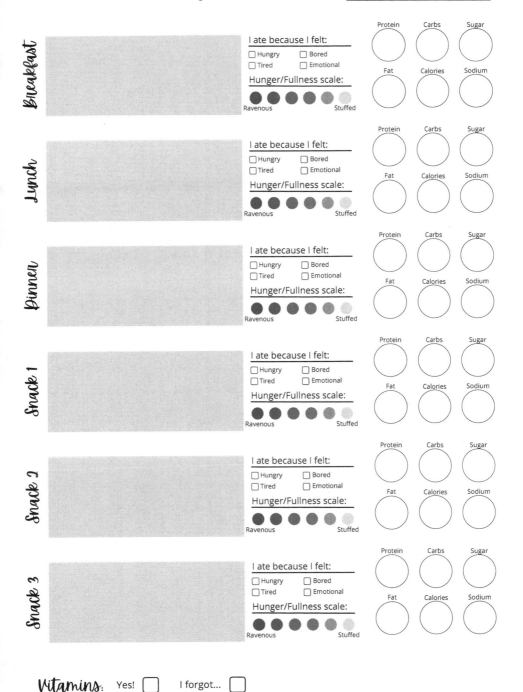

Breakfast

I ate because I felt:
- ☐ Hungry
- ☐ Tired
- ☐ Bored
- ☐ Emotional

Hunger/Fullness scale:
Ravenous ●●●●●○ Stuffed

Protein | Carbs | Sugar
Fat | Calories | Sodium

Lunch

I ate because I felt:
- ☐ Hungry
- ☐ Tired
- ☐ Bored
- ☐ Emotional

Hunger/Fullness scale:
Ravenous ●●●●●○ Stuffed

Protein | Carbs | Sugar
Fat | Calories | Sodium

Dinner

I ate because I felt:
- ☐ Hungry
- ☐ Tired
- ☐ Bored
- ☐ Emotional

Hunger/Fullness scale:
Ravenous ●●●●●○ Stuffed

Protein | Carbs | Sugar
Fat | Calories | Sodium

Snack 1

I ate because I felt:
- ☐ Hungry
- ☐ Tired
- ☐ Bored
- ☐ Emotional

Hunger/Fullness scale:
Ravenous ●●●●●○ Stuffed

Protein | Carbs | Sugar
Fat | Calories | Sodium

Snack 2

I ate because I felt:
- ☐ Hungry
- ☐ Tired
- ☐ Bored
- ☐ Emotional

Hunger/Fullness scale:
Ravenous ●●●●●○ Stuffed

Protein | Carbs | Sugar
Fat | Calories | Sodium

Snack 3

I ate because I felt:
- ☐ Hungry
- ☐ Tired
- ☐ Bored
- ☐ Emotional

Hunger/Fullness scale:
Ravenous ●●●●●○ Stuffed

Protein | Carbs | Sugar
Fat | Calories | Sodium

Vitamins: Yes! ☐   I forgot... ☐

Daily Planner

Sunday

Daily tasks:

♡ ....
♡ ....
♡ ....
♡ ....
♡ ....

My mood:

☹ ☹ ☺ ☺ ☺

Hours of sleep:

2   3   4   5   6   7   8   9   10   11   12
☐ ☐ ☐ ☐ ☐ ☐ ☐ ☐ ☐ ☐ ☐

Today's affirmation:

....
....

Notes:

Daily schedule:

8:00	
9:00	
10:00	
11:00	
12:00	
1:00	
2:00	
3:00	
4:00	
5:00	
6:00	
7:00	
8:00	
9:00	
10:00	

Food Diary

Breakfast

I ate because I felt:

- [ ] Hungry
- [ ] Tired
- [ ] Bored
- [ ] Emotional

Hunger/Fullness scale:

Ravenous ●●●●●○ Stuffed

Protein | Carbs | Sugar
Fat | Calories | Sodium

Lunch

I ate because I felt:

- [ ] Hungry
- [ ] Tired
- [ ] Bored
- [ ] Emotional

Hunger/Fullness scale:

Ravenous ●●●●●○ Stuffed

Protein | Carbs | Sugar
Fat | Calories | Sodium

Dinner

I ate because I felt:

- [ ] Hungry
- [ ] Tired
- [ ] Bored
- [ ] Emotional

Hunger/Fullness scale:

Ravenous ●●●●●○ Stuffed

Protein | Carbs | Sugar
Fat | Calories | Sodium

Snack 1

I ate because I felt:

- [ ] Hungry
- [ ] Tired
- [ ] Bored
- [ ] Emotional

Hunger/Fullness scale:

Ravenous ●●●●●○ Stuffed

Protein | Carbs | Sugar
Fat | Calories | Sodium

Snack 2

I ate because I felt:

- [ ] Hungry
- [ ] Tired
- [ ] Bored
- [ ] Emotional

Hunger/Fullness scale:

Ravenous ●●●●●○ Stuffed

Protein | Carbs | Sugar
Fat | Calories | Sodium

Snack 3

I ate because I felt:

- [ ] Hungry
- [ ] Tired
- [ ] Bored
- [ ] Emotional

Hunger/Fullness scale:

Ravenous ●●●●●○ Stuffed

Protein | Carbs | Sugar
Fat | Calories | Sodium

Vitamins: Yes! [ ] I forgot... [ ]

Hydration Tracker Week 5 _____

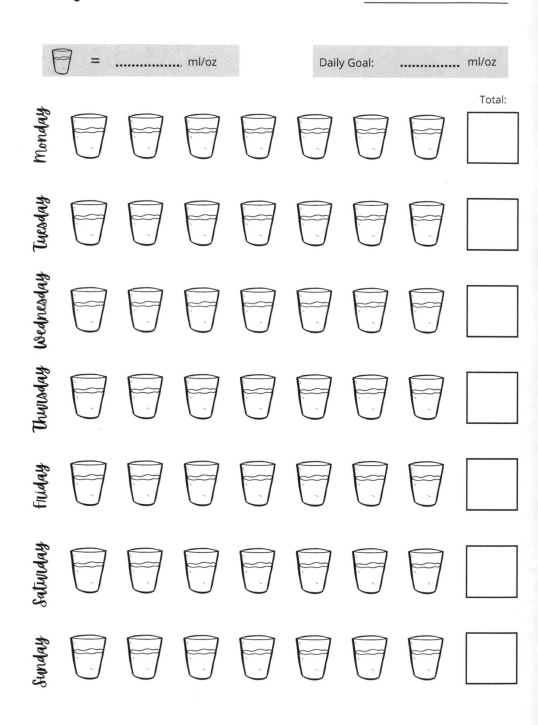

= .... ml/oz   Daily Goal: .... ml/oz

Monday   Total:

Tuesday

Wednesday

Thursday

Friday

Saturday

Sunday

Meal Planner

Week 5

Meals:

Monday

Tuesday

Wednesday

Thursday

Friday

Saturday

Sunday

Grocery List:

♡ ....
♡ ....
♡ ....
♡ ....
♡ ....
♡ ....
♡ ....
♡ ....
♡ ....
♡ ....
♡ ....
♡ ....
♡ ....
♡ ....
♡ ....
♡ ....
♡ ....
♡ ....
♡ ....
♡ ....
♡ ....
♡ ....

Activity Tracker

Daily Target: .... minutes

Minutes:

Monday
···
···

Tuesday
···
···

Wednesday
···
···

Thursday
···
···

Friday
···
···

Saturday
···
···

Sunday
···
···

Habit Tracker

Habit	MON	TUE	WED	THU	FRI	SAT	SUN
_____	○	○	○	○	○	○	○
_____	○	○	○	○	○	○	○
_____	○	○	○	○	○	○	○
_____	○	○	○	○	○	○	○
_____	○	○	○	○	○	○	○
_____	○	○	○	○	○	○	○
_____	○	○	○	○	○	○	○
_____	○	○	○	○	○	○	○
_____	○	○	○	○	○	○	○
_____	○	○	○	○	○	○	○
_____	○	○	○	○	○	○	○
_____	○	○	○	○	○	○	○
_____	○	○	○	○	○	○	○
_____	○	○	○	○	○	○	○
_____	○	○	○	○	○	○	○
_____	○	○	○	○	○	○	○
_____	○	○	○	○	○	○	○

Notes:

....

....

....

Bariatric surgery isn't cheating.

Weigh-In

Highest Weight

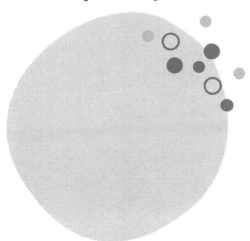

Weight Last Week

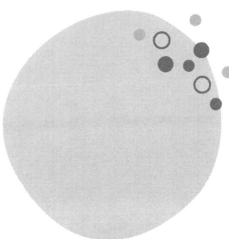

Weekly Weight Loss +/-

Current Weight

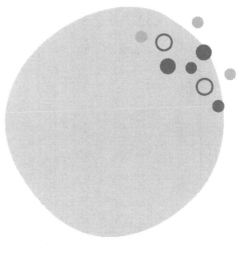

Notes:

Measurements

	Highest	Last Week	This Week	Lost
Neck				
Shoulders				
Chest				
Right Arm				
Left Arm				
Waist				
Hips				
Right Thigh				
Left Thigh				
Right Calf				
Left Calf				

Notes:

....

....

....

Progress Picture

Worthy Then

Worthy Now

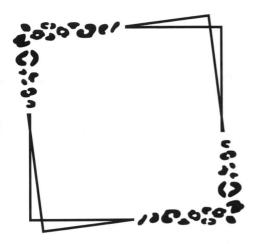

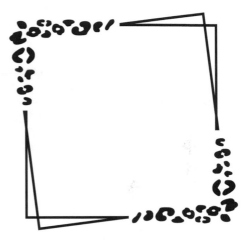

Date: ....

Weight: ....

Date: ....

Weight: ....

Describe how you felt in both pictures:

....

....

....

....

Reflection

Skills I have worked on this week:

....

....

....

....

I still need to be more mindful of:

....

....

....

....

I am thankful for:

....

....

....

....

Next week I will focus more on:

....

....

....

Brain Dump

What's on your mind?

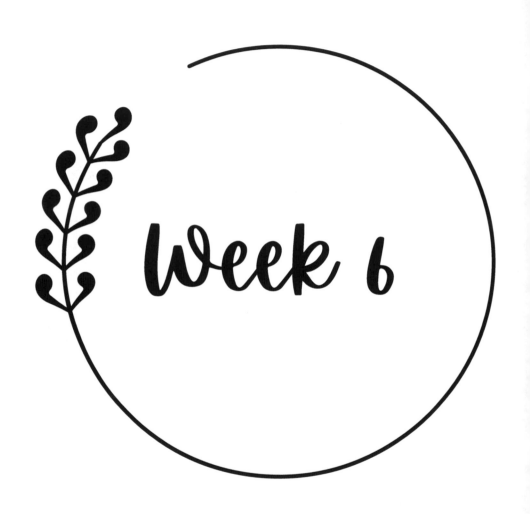

Week 6

Weekly Planner

Priorities:

♡ ....
♡ ....
♡ ....
♡ ....
♡ ....

To do:

☐ ....
☐ ....
☐ ....
☐ ....
☐ ....
☐ ....
☐ ....
☐ ....
☐ ....
☐ ....

Notes:

Monday

Tuesday

Wednesday

Thursday

Friday

Saturday

Sunday

Daily Planner

Daily tasks:

♡ ....
♡ ....
♡ ....
♡ ....
♡ ....

My mood:

☹ 😦 😐 🙂 😃

Hours of sleep:

2	3	4	5	6	7	8	9	10	11	12
☐	☐	☐	☐	☐	☐	☐	☐	☐	☐	☐

Today's affirmation:

....

....

Notes:

Daily schedule:

8:00	
9:00	
10:00	
11:00	
12:00	
1:00	
2:00	
3:00	
4:00	
5:00	
6:00	
7:00	
8:00	
9:00	
10:00	

141

Food Diary

Breakfast

I ate because I felt:

☐ Hungry   ☐ Bored
☐ Tired   ☐ Emotional

Hunger/Fullness scale:

Ravenous ●●●●●○ Stuffed

Protein   Carbs   Sugar
○   ○   ○

Fat   Calories Sodium
○   ○   ○

Lunch

I ate because I felt:

☐ Hungry   ☐ Bored
☐ Tired   ☐ Emotional

Hunger/Fullness scale:

Ravenous ●●●●●○ Stuffed

Protein   Carbs   Sugar
○   ○   ○

Fat   Calories Sodium
○   ○   ○

Dinner

I ate because I felt:

☐ Hungry   ☐ Bored
☐ Tired   ☐ Emotional

Hunger/Fullness scale:

Ravenous ●●●●●○ Stuffed

Protein   Carbs   Sugar
○   ○   ○

Fat   Calories Sodium
○   ○   ○

Snack 1

I ate because I felt:

☐ Hungry   ☐ Bored
☐ Tired   ☐ Emotional

Hunger/Fullness scale:

Ravenous ●●●●●○ Stuffed

Protein   Carbs   Sugar
○   ○   ○

Fat   Calories Sodium
○   ○   ○

Snack 2

I ate because I felt:

☐ Hungry   ☐ Bored
☐ Tired   ☐ Emotional

Hunger/Fullness scale:

Ravenous ●●●●●○ Stuffed

Protein   Carbs   Sugar
○   ○   ○

Fat   Calories Sodium
○   ○   ○

Snack 3

I ate because I felt:

☐ Hungry   ☐ Bored
☐ Tired   ☐ Emotional

Hunger/Fullness scale:

Ravenous ●●●●●○ Stuffed

Protein   Carbs   Sugar
○   ○   ○

Fat   Calories Sodium
○   ○   ○

Vitamins: Yes! ☐   I forgot... ☐

Daily Planner

Daily tasks:

♡ ....
♡ ....
♡ ....
♡ ....
♡ ....

My mood:

☹ ☹ 😐 ☺ 😃

Hours of sleep:

2 3 4 5 6 7 8 9 10 11 12
☐ ☐ ☐ ☐ ☐ ☐ ☐ ☐ ☐ ☐ ☐

Today's affirmation:

....
....

Notes:

Daily schedule:

Time	
8.00	
9.00	
10.00	
11.00	
12.00	
1.00	
2.00	
3.00	
4.00	
5.00	
6.00	
7.00	
8.00	
9.00	
10.00	

Food Diary

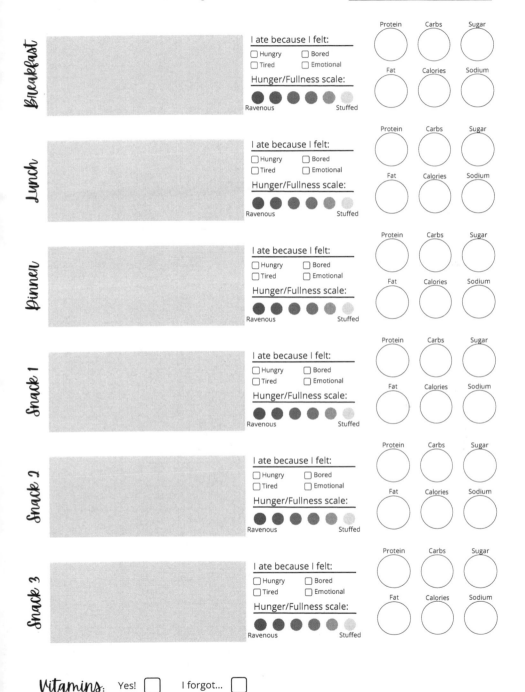

Breakfast

I ate because I felt:
- ☐ Hungry
- ☐ Tired
- ☐ Bored
- ☐ Emotional

Hunger/Fullness scale:

Ravenous ●●●●●○ Stuffed

Protein | Carbs | Sugar
Fat | Calories | Sodium

Lunch

I ate because I felt:
- ☐ Hungry
- ☐ Tired
- ☐ Bored
- ☐ Emotional

Hunger/Fullness scale:

Ravenous ●●●●●○ Stuffed

Protein | Carbs | Sugar
Fat | Calories | Sodium

Dinner

I ate because I felt:
- ☐ Hungry
- ☐ Tired
- ☐ Bored
- ☐ Emotional

Hunger/Fullness scale:

Ravenous ●●●●●○ Stuffed

Protein | Carbs | Sugar
Fat | Calories | Sodium

Snack 1

I ate because I felt:
- ☐ Hungry
- ☐ Tired
- ☐ Bored
- ☐ Emotional

Hunger/Fullness scale:

Ravenous ●●●●●○ Stuffed

Protein | Carbs | Sugar
Fat | Calories | Sodium

Snack 2

I ate because I felt:
- ☐ Hungry
- ☐ Tired
- ☐ Bored
- ☐ Emotional

Hunger/Fullness scale:

Ravenous ●●●●●○ Stuffed

Protein | Carbs | Sugar
Fat | Calories | Sodium

Snack 3

I ate because I felt:
- ☐ Hungry
- ☐ Tired
- ☐ Bored
- ☐ Emotional

Hunger/Fullness scale:

Ravenous ●●●●●○ Stuffed

Protein | Carbs | Sugar
Fat | Calories | Sodium

Vitamins: Yes! ☐   I forgot... ☐

144

Daily Planner

Daily tasks:

♡ ....
♡ ....
♡ ....
♡ ....
♡ ....

My mood:

☹ ☹ 😐 🙂 😃

Hours of sleep:

2 3 4 5 6 7 8 9 10 11 12
☐ ☐ ☐ ☐ ☐ ☐ ☐ ☐ ☐   ☐   ☐

Today's affirmation:

....

....

Notes:

Daily schedule:

8.00	
9.00	
10.00	
11.00	
12.00	
1.00	
2.00	
3.00	
4.00	
5.00	
6.00	
7.00	
8.00	
9.00	
10.00	

Food Diary

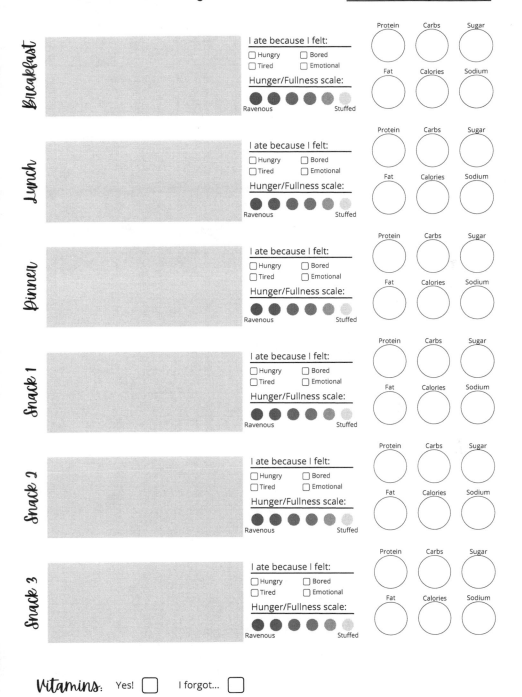

Breakfast

I ate because I felt:
- ☐ Hungry
- ☐ Tired
- ☐ Bored
- ☐ Emotional

Hunger/Fullness scale:

Ravenous ●●●●●○ Stuffed

Protein | Carbs | Sugar

Fat | Calories | Sodium

Lunch

I ate because I felt:
- ☐ Hungry
- ☐ Tired
- ☐ Bored
- ☐ Emotional

Hunger/Fullness scale:

Ravenous ●●●●●○ Stuffed

Protein | Carbs | Sugar

Fat | Calories | Sodium

Dinner

I ate because I felt:
- ☐ Hungry
- ☐ Tired
- ☐ Bored
- ☐ Emotional

Hunger/Fullness scale:

Ravenous ●●●●●○ Stuffed

Protein | Carbs | Sugar

Fat | Calories | Sodium

Snack 1

I ate because I felt:
- ☐ Hungry
- ☐ Tired
- ☐ Bored
- ☐ Emotional

Hunger/Fullness scale:

Ravenous ●●●●●○ Stuffed

Protein | Carbs | Sugar

Fat | Calories | Sodium

Snack 2

I ate because I felt:
- ☐ Hungry
- ☐ Tired
- ☐ Bored
- ☐ Emotional

Hunger/Fullness scale:

Ravenous ●●●●●○ Stuffed

Protein | Carbs | Sugar

Fat | Calories | Sodium

Snack 3

I ate because I felt:
- ☐ Hungry
- ☐ Tired
- ☐ Bored
- ☐ Emotional

Hunger/Fullness scale:

Ravenous ●●●●●○ Stuffed

Protein | Carbs | Sugar

Fat | Calories | Sodium

Vitamins: Yes! ☐   I forgot... ☐

Daily Planner

Daily tasks:

- ♡ ....
- ♡ ....
- ♡ ....
- ♡ ....
- ♡ ....

My mood:

☹ 😦 😐 🙂 😃

Hours of sleep:

2	3	4	5	6	7	8	9	10	11	12
☐	☐	☐	☐	☐	☐	☐	☐	☐	☐	☐

Today's affirmation:

....

....

Notes:

Daily schedule:

8.00	
9.00	
10.00	
11.00	
12.00	
1.00	
2.00	
3.00	
4.00	
5.00	
6.00	
7.00	
8.00	
9.00	
10.00	

147

Food Diary

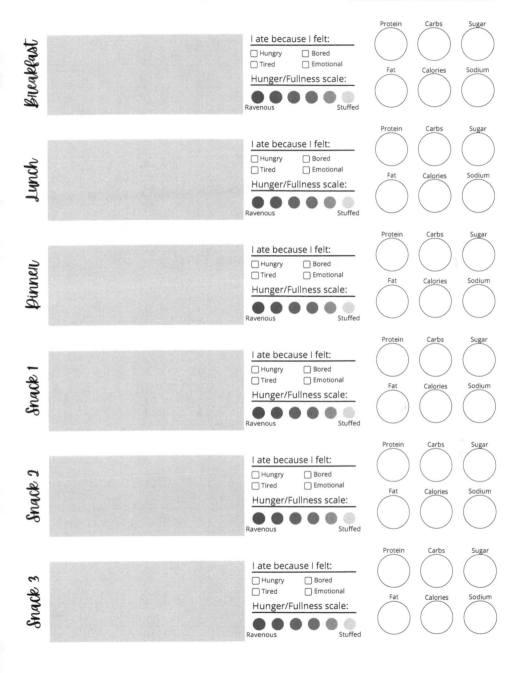

Breakfast

I ate because I felt:
- ☐ Hungry
- ☐ Tired
- ☐ Bored
- ☐ Emotional

Hunger/Fullness scale:
Ravenous ●●●●●○ Stuffed

Protein | Carbs | Sugar
Fat | Calories | Sodium

Lunch

I ate because I felt:
- ☐ Hungry
- ☐ Tired
- ☐ Bored
- ☐ Emotional

Hunger/Fullness scale:
Ravenous ●●●●●○ Stuffed

Protein | Carbs | Sugar
Fat | Calories | Sodium

Dinner

I ate because I felt:
- ☐ Hungry
- ☐ Tired
- ☐ Bored
- ☐ Emotional

Hunger/Fullness scale:
Ravenous ●●●●●○ Stuffed

Protein | Carbs | Sugar
Fat | Calories | Sodium

Snack 1

I ate because I felt:
- ☐ Hungry
- ☐ Tired
- ☐ Bored
- ☐ Emotional

Hunger/Fullness scale:
Ravenous ●●●●●○ Stuffed

Protein | Carbs | Sugar
Fat | Calories | Sodium

Snack 2

I ate because I felt:
- ☐ Hungry
- ☐ Tired
- ☐ Bored
- ☐ Emotional

Hunger/Fullness scale:
Ravenous ●●●●●○ Stuffed

Protein | Carbs | Sugar
Fat | Calories | Sodium

Snack 3

I ate because I felt:
- ☐ Hungry
- ☐ Tired
- ☐ Bored
- ☐ Emotional

Hunger/Fullness scale:
Ravenous ●●●●●○ Stuffed

Protein | Carbs | Sugar
Fat | Calories | Sodium

Vitamins: Yes! ☐   I forgot... ☐

Daily Planner

Daily tasks:

♡ ....
♡ ....
♡ ....
♡ ....
♡ ....

My mood:

☹ ☹ 😐 🙂 😀

Hours of sleep:

2	3	4	5	6	7	8	9	10	11	12
☐	☐	☐	☐	☐	☐	☐	☐	☐	☐	☐

Today's affirmation:

....

....

Notes:

Daily schedule:

8:00	
9:00	
10:00	
11:00	
12:00	
1:00	
2:00	
3:00	
4:00	
5:00	
6:00	
7:00	
8:00	
9:00	
10:00	

Food Diary

Breakfast

I ate because I felt:
- [ ] Hungry
- [ ] Tired
- [ ] Bored
- [ ] Emotional

Hunger/Fullness scale:

Ravenous ●●●●●○ Stuffed

Protein | Carbs | Sugar
Fat | Calories | Sodium

Lunch

I ate because I felt:
- [ ] Hungry
- [ ] Tired
- [ ] Bored
- [ ] Emotional

Hunger/Fullness scale:

Ravenous ●●●●●○ Stuffed

Protein | Carbs | Sugar
Fat | Calories | Sodium

Dinner

I ate because I felt:
- [ ] Hungry
- [ ] Tired
- [ ] Bored
- [ ] Emotional

Hunger/Fullness scale:

Ravenous ●●●●●○ Stuffed

Protein | Carbs | Sugar
Fat | Calories | Sodium

Snack 1

I ate because I felt:
- [ ] Hungry
- [ ] Tired
- [ ] Bored
- [ ] Emotional

Hunger/Fullness scale:

Ravenous ●●●●●○ Stuffed

Protein | Carbs | Sugar
Fat | Calories | Sodium

Snack 2

I ate because I felt:
- [ ] Hungry
- [ ] Tired
- [ ] Bored
- [ ] Emotional

Hunger/Fullness scale:

Ravenous ●●●●●○ Stuffed

Protein | Carbs | Sugar
Fat | Calories | Sodium

Snack 3

I ate because I felt:
- [ ] Hungry
- [ ] Tired
- [ ] Bored
- [ ] Emotional

Hunger/Fullness scale:

Ravenous ●●●●●○ Stuffed

Protein | Carbs | Sugar
Fat | Calories | Sodium

Vitamins: Yes! [ ]   I forgot... [ ]

150

Daily Planner

Saturday

Daily tasks:

♡ ....
♡ ....
♡ ....
♡ ....
♡ ....

My mood:

☹ ☹ 😐 🙂 😃

Hours of sleep:

2 3 4 5 6 7 8 9 10 11 12
☐ ☐ ☐ ☐ ☐ ☐ ☐ ☐ ☐   ☐   ☐

Today's affirmation:

....

....

Notes:

Daily schedule:

8.00	
9.00	
10.00	
11.00	
12.00	
1.00	
2.00	
3.00	
4.00	
5.00	
6.00	
7.00	
8.00	
9.00	
10.00	

Food Diary

Breakfast

I ate because I felt:

☐ Hungry   ☐ Bored
☐ Tired   ☐ Emotional

Hunger/Fullness scale:

Ravenous ●●●●●○ Stuffed

Protein   Carbs   Sugar
○   ○   ○

Fat   Calories Sodium
○   ○   ○

Lunch

I ate because I felt:

☐ Hungry   ☐ Bored
☐ Tired   ☐ Emotional

Hunger/Fullness scale:

Ravenous ●●●●●○ Stuffed

Protein   Carbs   Sugar
○   ○   ○

Fat   Calories Sodium
○   ○   ○

Dinner

I ate because I felt:

☐ Hungry   ☐ Bored
☐ Tired   ☐ Emotional

Hunger/Fullness scale:

Ravenous ●●●●●○ Stuffed

Protein   Carbs   Sugar
○   ○   ○

Fat   Calories Sodium
○   ○   ○

Snack 1

I ate because I felt:

☐ Hungry   ☐ Bored
☐ Tired   ☐ Emotional

Hunger/Fullness scale:

Ravenous ●●●●●○ Stuffed

Protein   Carbs   Sugar
○   ○   ○

Fat   Calories Sodium
○   ○   ○

Snack 2

I ate because I felt:

☐ Hungry   ☐ Bored
☐ Tired   ☐ Emotional

Hunger/Fullness scale:

Ravenous ●●●●●○ Stuffed

Protein   Carbs   Sugar
○   ○   ○

Fat   Calories Sodium
○   ○   ○

Snack 3

I ate because I felt:

☐ Hungry   ☐ Bored
☐ Tired   ☐ Emotional

Hunger/Fullness scale:

Ravenous ●●●●●○ Stuffed

Protein   Carbs   Sugar
○   ○   ○

Fat   Calories Sodium
○   ○   ○

Vitamins: Yes! ☐   I forgot... ☐

Daily Planner

Daily tasks:

♡ ....
♡ ....
♡ ....
♡ ....
♡ ....

My mood:

☹ ☹ 😐 🙂 😃

Hours of sleep:

2	3	4	5	6	7	8	9	10	11	12
☐	☐	☐	☐	☐	☐	☐	☐	☐	☐	☐

Today's affirmation:

....

....

Notes:

Daily schedule:

8.00	
9.00	
10.00	
11.00	
12.00	
1.00	
2.00	
3.00	
4.00	
5.00	
6.00	
7.00	
8.00	
9.00	
10.00	

153

Food Diary

Sunday _____

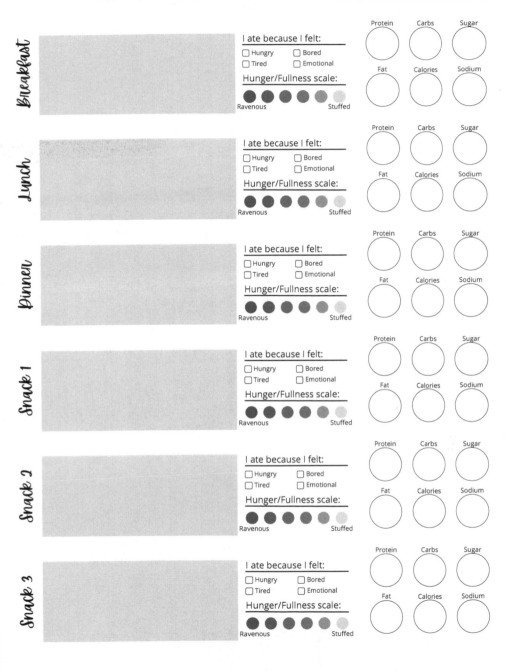

Breakfast

I ate because I felt:
- [ ] Hungry
- [ ] Bored
- [ ] Tired
- [ ] Emotional

Hunger/Fullness scale:

Ravenous ●●●●●● Stuffed

Protein ○ Carbs ○ Sugar ○
Fat ○ Calories ○ Sodium ○

Lunch

I ate because I felt:
- [ ] Hungry
- [ ] Bored
- [ ] Tired
- [ ] Emotional

Hunger/Fullness scale:

Ravenous ●●●●●● Stuffed

Protein ○ Carbs ○ Sugar ○
Fat ○ Calories ○ Sodium ○

Dinner

I ate because I felt:
- [ ] Hungry
- [ ] Bored
- [ ] Tired
- [ ] Emotional

Hunger/Fullness scale:

Ravenous ●●●●●● Stuffed

Protein ○ Carbs ○ Sugar ○
Fat ○ Calories ○ Sodium ○

Snack 1

I ate because I felt:
- [ ] Hungry
- [ ] Bored
- [ ] Tired
- [ ] Emotional

Hunger/Fullness scale:

Ravenous ●●●●●● Stuffed

Protein ○ Carbs ○ Sugar ○
Fat ○ Calories ○ Sodium ○

Snack 2

I ate because I felt:
- [ ] Hungry
- [ ] Bored
- [ ] Tired
- [ ] Emotional

Hunger/Fullness scale:

Ravenous ●●●●●● Stuffed

Protein ○ Carbs ○ Sugar ○
Fat ○ Calories ○ Sodium ○

Snack 3

I ate because I felt:
- [ ] Hungry
- [ ] Bored
- [ ] Tired
- [ ] Emotional

Hunger/Fullness scale:

Ravenous ●●●●●● Stuffed

Protein ○ Carbs ○ Sugar ○
Fat ○ Calories ○ Sodium ○

Vitamins: Yes! [ ]   I forgot... [ ]

154

Hydration Tracker Week 6

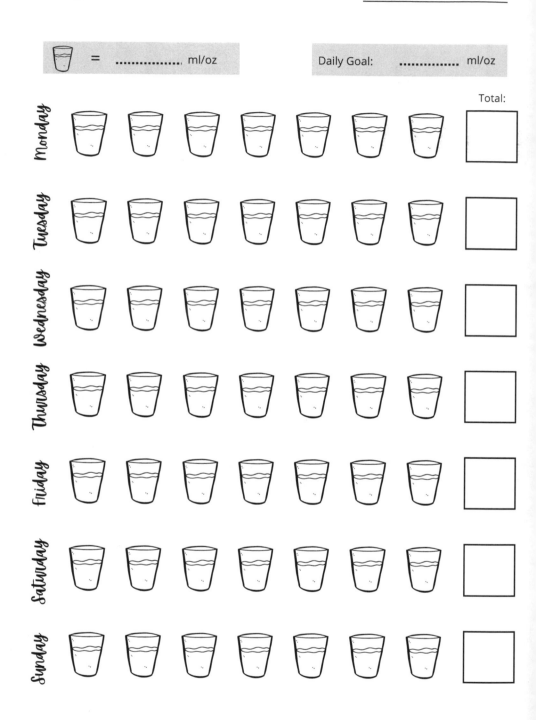

Meal Planner

Meals: | Grocery List:

Monday

Tuesday

Wednesday

Thursday

friday

Saturday

Sunday

Grocery List:
- ♡ ....
- ♡ ....
- ♡ ....
- ♡ ....
- ♡ ....
- ♡ ....
- ♡ ....
- ♡ ....
- ♡ ....
- ♡ ....
- ♡ ....
- ♡ ....
- ♡ ....
- ♡ ....
- ♡ ....
- ♡ ....
- ♡ ....
- ♡ ....
- ♡ ....
- ♡ ....
- ♡ ....
- ♡ ....

Activity Tracker

Week 6

Daily Target: .... minutes

Minutes:

Monday

Tuesday

Wednesday

Thursday

Friday

Saturday

Sunday

Habit Tracker

Habit	MON	TUE	WED	THU	FRI	SAT	SUN
	○	○	○	○	○	○	○
	○	○	○	○	○	○	○
	○	○	○	○	○	○	○
	○	○	○	○	○	○	○
	○	○	○	○	○	○	○
	○	○	○	○	○	○	○
	○	○	○	○	○	○	○
	○	○	○	○	○	○	○
	○	○	○	○	○	○	○
	○	○	○	○	○	○	○
	○	○	○	○	○	○	○
	○	○	○	○	○	○	○
	○	○	○	○	○	○	○
	○	○	○	○	○	○	○
	○	○	○	○	○	○	○
	○	○	○	○	○	○	○
	○	○	○	○	○	○	○

Notes:

Removing or bypassing 80% of your stomach - requires 100% commitment.

Weigh-In

Highest Weight

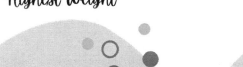

Weight Last Week

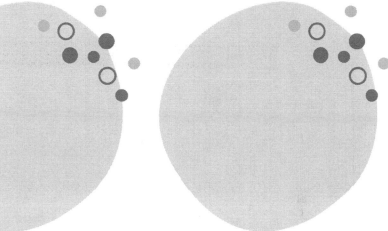

Weekly Weight Loss +/-

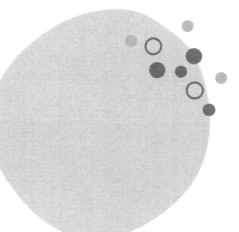

Current Weight

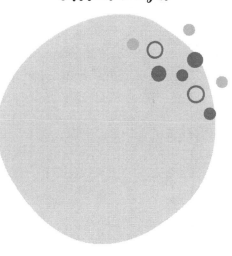

Notes:

....

....

Measurements

	Highest	Last Week	This Week	Lost
Neck				
Shoulders				
Chest				
Right Arm				
Left Arm				
Waist				
Hips				
Right Thigh				
Left Thigh				
Right Calf				
Left Calf				

Notes:

....

....

....

Progress Picture

Worthy Then

Worthy Now

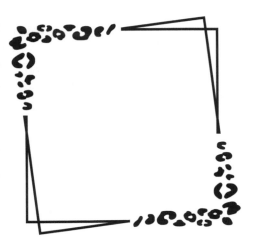
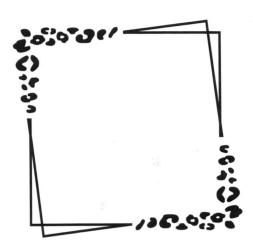

Date: ....

Weight: ....

Date: ....

Weight: ....

Describe how you felt in both pictures:

....

....

....

....

Reflection

Skills I have worked on this week:

....

....

....

....

I still need to be more mindful of:

....

....

....

....

I am thankful for:

....

....

....

....

Next week I will focus more on:

....

....

....

Brain Dump

What's on your mind?

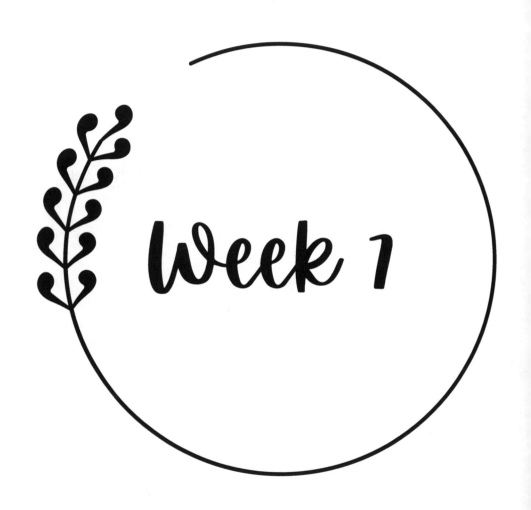

Weekly Planner

Priorities:

♡ ....
♡ ....
♡ ....
♡ ....
♡ ....

To do:

☐ ....
☐ ....
☐ ....
☐ ....
☐ ....
☐ ....
☐ ....
☐ ....
☐ ....
☐ ....
☐ ....

Notes:

Monday

Tuesday

Wednesday

Thursday

Friday

Saturday

Sunday

Daily Planner

Daily tasks:

♡ ....

♡ ....

♡ ....

♡ ....

♡ ....

My mood:

☹ ☹ 😐 🙂 😃

Hours of sleep:

2	3	4	5	6	7	8	9	10	11	12
☐	☐	☐	☐	☐	☐	☐	☐	☐	☐	☐

Today's affirmation:

....

....

Notes:

Daily schedule:

8.00	
9.00	
10.00	
11.00	
12.00	
1.00	
2.00	
3.00	
4.00	
5.00	
6.00	
7.00	
8.00	
9.00	
10.00	

Food Diary

Monday

Breakfast

I ate because I felt:
- [ ] Hungry
- [ ] Bored
- [ ] Tired
- [ ] Emotional

Hunger/Fullness scale:

Ravenous   Stuffed

Protein   Carbs   Sugar

Fat   Calories   Sodium

Lunch

I ate because I felt:
- [ ] Hungry
- [ ] Bored
- [ ] Tired
- [ ] Emotional

Hunger/Fullness scale:

Ravenous   Stuffed

Protein   Carbs   Sugar

Fat   Calories   Sodium

Dinner

I ate because I felt:
- [ ] Hungry
- [ ] Bored
- [ ] Tired
- [ ] Emotional

Hunger/Fullness scale:

Ravenous   Stuffed

Protein   Carbs   Sugar

Fat   Calories   Sodium

Snack 1

I ate because I felt:
- [ ] Hungry
- [ ] Bored
- [ ] Tired
- [ ] Emotional

Hunger/Fullness scale:

Ravenous   Stuffed

Protein   Carbs   Sugar

Fat   Calories   Sodium

Snack 2

I ate because I felt:
- [ ] Hungry
- [ ] Bored
- [ ] Tired
- [ ] Emotional

Hunger/Fullness scale:

Ravenous   Stuffed

Protein   Carbs   Sugar

Fat   Calories   Sodium

Snack 3

I ate because I felt:
- [ ] Hungry
- [ ] Bored
- [ ] Tired
- [ ] Emotional

Hunger/Fullness scale:

Ravenous   Stuffed

Protein   Carbs   Sugar

Fat   Calories   Sodium

Vitamins: Yes! [ ]   I forgot... [ ]

Daily Planner

Daily tasks:

♡ ....
♡ ....
♡ ....
♡ ....
♡ ....

My mood:

☹ ☹ 😐 🙂 😃

Hours of sleep:

2	3	4	5	6	7	8	9	10	11	12
☐	☐	☐	☐	☐	☐	☐	☐	☐	☐	☐

Today's affirmation:

....

....

Notes:

Daily schedule:

8:00	
9:00	
10:00	
11:00	
12:00	
1:00	
2:00	
3:00	
4:00	
5:00	
6:00	
7:00	
8:00	
9:00	
10:00	

169

Food Diary

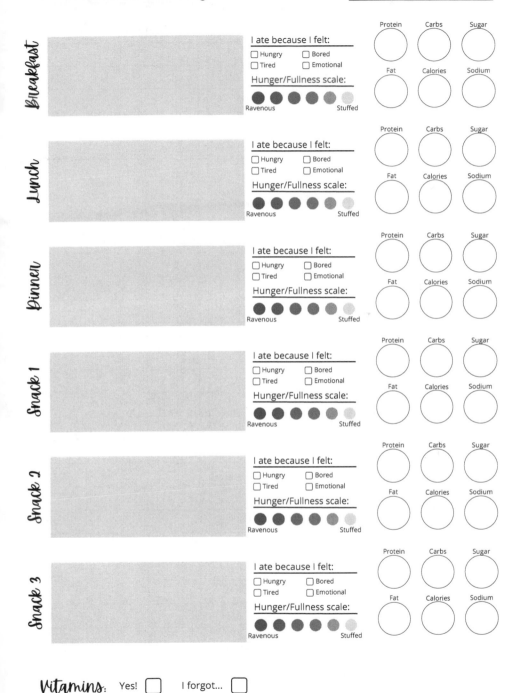

Breakfast

I ate because I felt:
- [ ] Hungry
- [ ] Tired
- [ ] Bored
- [ ] Emotional

Hunger/Fullness scale:
Ravenous ●●●●●○ Stuffed

Protein Carbs Sugar
Fat Calories Sodium

Lunch

I ate because I felt:
- [ ] Hungry
- [ ] Tired
- [ ] Bored
- [ ] Emotional

Hunger/Fullness scale:
Ravenous ●●●●●○ Stuffed

Protein Carbs Sugar
Fat Calories Sodium

Dinner

I ate because I felt:
- [ ] Hungry
- [ ] Tired
- [ ] Bored
- [ ] Emotional

Hunger/Fullness scale:
Ravenous ●●●●●○ Stuffed

Protein Carbs Sugar
Fat Calories Sodium

Snack 1

I ate because I felt:
- [ ] Hungry
- [ ] Tired
- [ ] Bored
- [ ] Emotional

Hunger/Fullness scale:
Ravenous ●●●●●○ Stuffed

Protein Carbs Sugar
Fat Calories Sodium

Snack 2

I ate because I felt:
- [ ] Hungry
- [ ] Tired
- [ ] Bored
- [ ] Emotional

Hunger/Fullness scale:
Ravenous ●●●●●○ Stuffed

Protein Carbs Sugar
Fat Calories Sodium

Snack 3

I ate because I felt:
- [ ] Hungry
- [ ] Tired
- [ ] Bored
- [ ] Emotional

Hunger/Fullness scale:
Ravenous ●●●●●○ Stuffed

Protein Carbs Sugar
Fat Calories Sodium

Vitamins: Yes! [ ]   I forgot... [ ]

Daily Planner

Daily tasks:

♡ ....
♡ ....
♡ ....
♡ ....
♡ ....

My mood:

😢 😦 😐 🙂 😃

Hours of sleep:

2	3	4	5	6	7	8	9	10	11	12
☐	☐	☐	☐	☐	☐	☐	☐	☐	☐	☐

Today's affirmation:

....

....

Notes:

Daily schedule:

8:00	
9:00	
10:00	
11:00	
12:00	
1:00	
2:00	
3:00	
4:00	
5:00	
6:00	
7:00	
8:00	
9:00	
10:00	

Food Diary

Breakfast

I ate because I felt:
- [ ] Hungry
- [ ] Bored
- [ ] Tired
- [ ] Emotional

Hunger/Fullness scale:

Ravenous ●●●●●● Stuffed

Protein Carbs Sugar
Fat Calories Sodium

Lunch

I ate because I felt:
- [ ] Hungry
- [ ] Bored
- [ ] Tired
- [ ] Emotional

Hunger/Fullness scale:

Ravenous ●●●●●● Stuffed

Protein Carbs Sugar
Fat Calories Sodium

Dinner

I ate because I felt:
- [ ] Hungry
- [ ] Bored
- [ ] Tired
- [ ] Emotional

Hunger/Fullness scale:

Ravenous ●●●●●● Stuffed

Protein Carbs Sugar
Fat Calories Sodium

Snack 1

I ate because I felt:
- [ ] Hungry
- [ ] Bored
- [ ] Tired
- [ ] Emotional

Hunger/Fullness scale:

Ravenous ●●●●●● Stuffed

Protein Carbs Sugar
Fat Calories Sodium

Snack 2

I ate because I felt:
- [ ] Hungry
- [ ] Bored
- [ ] Tired
- [ ] Emotional

Hunger/Fullness scale:

Ravenous ●●●●●● Stuffed

Protein Carbs Sugar
Fat Calories Sodium

Snack 3

I ate because I felt:
- [ ] Hungry
- [ ] Bored
- [ ] Tired
- [ ] Emotional

Hunger/Fullness scale:

Ravenous ●●●●●● Stuffed

Protein Carbs Sugar
Fat Calories Sodium

Vitamins: Yes! [ ]   I forgot... [ ]

Daily Planner

Daily tasks:

♡ ....
♡ ....
♡ ....
♡ ....
♡ ....

My mood:

☹ 😦 😐 🙂 😃

Hours of sleep:

2 3 4 5 6 7 8 9 10 11 12
☐ ☐ ☐ ☐ ☐ ☐ ☐ ☐ ☐ ☐ ☐

Today's affirmation:

....

....

Notes:

Daily schedule:

8:00	
9:00	
10:00	
11:00	
12:00	
1:00	
2:00	
3:00	
4:00	
5:00	
6:00	
7:00	
8:00	
9:00	
10:00	

Food Diary

Breakfast

I ate because I felt:
- [ ] Hungry
- [ ] Tired
- [ ] Bored
- [ ] Emotional

Hunger/Fullness scale:

Ravenous ●●●●● Stuffed

Protein · Carbs · Sugar

Fat · Calories · Sodium

Lunch

I ate because I felt:
- [ ] Hungry
- [ ] Tired
- [ ] Bored
- [ ] Emotional

Hunger/Fullness scale:

Ravenous ●●●●● Stuffed

Protein · Carbs · Sugar

Fat · Calories · Sodium

Dinner

I ate because I felt:
- [ ] Hungry
- [ ] Tired
- [ ] Bored
- [ ] Emotional

Hunger/Fullness scale:

Ravenous ●●●●● Stuffed

Protein · Carbs · Sugar

Fat · Calories · Sodium

Snack 1

I ate because I felt:
- [ ] Hungry
- [ ] Tired
- [ ] Bored
- [ ] Emotional

Hunger/Fullness scale:

Ravenous ●●●●● Stuffed

Protein · Carbs · Sugar

Fat · Calories · Sodium

Snack 2

I ate because I felt:
- [ ] Hungry
- [ ] Tired
- [ ] Bored
- [ ] Emotional

Hunger/Fullness scale:

Ravenous ●●●●● Stuffed

Protein · Carbs · Sugar

Fat · Calories · Sodium

Snack 3

I ate because I felt:
- [ ] Hungry
- [ ] Tired
- [ ] Bored
- [ ] Emotional

Hunger/Fullness scale:

Ravenous ●●●●● Stuffed

Protein · Carbs · Sugar

Fat · Calories · Sodium

Vitamins: Yes! [ ]   I forgot... [ ]

Daily Planner

Friday

Daily tasks:

♡ ....
♡ ....
♡ ....
♡ ....
♡ ....

My mood:

😢 😟 😐 🙂 😃

Hours of sleep:

2	3	4	5	6	7	8	9	10	11	12
☐	☐	☐	☐	☐	☐	☐	☐	☐	☐	☐

Today's affirmation:

....

....

Notes:

Daily schedule:

8:00	
9:00	
10:00	
11:00	
12:00	
1:00	
2:00	
3:00	
4:00	
5:00	
6:00	
7:00	
8:00	
9:00	
10:00	

Food Diary

Breakfast

I ate because I felt:

☐ Hungry ☐ Bored
☐ Tired ☐ Emotional

Hunger/Fullness scale:

Ravenous ●●●●●● Stuffed

Protein Carbs Sugar

Fat Calories Sodium

Lunch

I ate because I felt:

☐ Hungry ☐ Bored
☐ Tired ☐ Emotional

Hunger/Fullness scale:

Ravenous ●●●●●● Stuffed

Protein Carbs Sugar

Fat Calories Sodium

Dinner

I ate because I felt:

☐ Hungry ☐ Bored
☐ Tired ☐ Emotional

Hunger/Fullness scale:

Ravenous ●●●●●● Stuffed

Protein Carbs Sugar

Fat Calories Sodium

Snack 1

I ate because I felt:

☐ Hungry ☐ Bored
☐ Tired ☐ Emotional

Hunger/Fullness scale:

Ravenous ●●●●●● Stuffed

Protein Carbs Sugar

Fat Calories Sodium

Snack 2

I ate because I felt:

☐ Hungry ☐ Bored
☐ Tired ☐ Emotional

Hunger/Fullness scale:

Ravenous ●●●●●● Stuffed

Protein Carbs Sugar

Fat Calories Sodium

Snack 3

I ate because I felt:

☐ Hungry ☐ Bored
☐ Tired ☐ Emotional

Hunger/Fullness scale:

Ravenous ●●●●●● Stuffed

Protein Carbs Sugar

Fat Calories Sodium

Vitamins: Yes! ☐   I forgot... ☐

Daily Planner

Daily tasks:

♡ ....
♡ ....
♡ ....
♡ ....
♡ ....

My mood:

☹ ☹ 😐 ☺ 😄

Hours of sleep:

2	3	4	5	6	7	8	9	10	11	12
☐	☐	☐	☐	☐	☐	☐	☐	☐	☐	☐

Today's affirmation:

....

....

Notes:

Daily schedule:

8:00	
9:00	
10:00	
11:00	
12:00	
1:00	
2:00	
3:00	
4:00	
5:00	
6:00	
7:00	
8:00	
9:00	
10:00	

Food Diary

Breakfast

I ate because I felt:
- [ ] Hungry
- [ ] Tired
- [ ] Bored
- [ ] Emotional

Hunger/Fullness scale:

Ravenous ●●●●● Stuffed

Protein

Carbs

Sugar

Fat

Calories

Sodium

Lunch

I ate because I felt:
- [ ] Hungry
- [ ] Tired
- [ ] Bored
- [ ] Emotional

Hunger/Fullness scale:

Ravenous ●●●●● Stuffed

Protein

Carbs

Sugar

Fat

Calories

Sodium

Dinner

I ate because I felt:
- [ ] Hungry
- [ ] Tired
- [ ] Bored
- [ ] Emotional

Hunger/Fullness scale:

Ravenous ●●●●● Stuffed

Protein

Carbs

Sugar

Fat

Calories

Sodium

Snack 1

I ate because I felt:
- [ ] Hungry
- [ ] Tired
- [ ] Bored
- [ ] Emotional

Hunger/Fullness scale:

Ravenous ●●●●● Stuffed

Protein

Carbs

Sugar

Fat

Calories

Sodium

Snack 2

I ate because I felt:
- [ ] Hungry
- [ ] Tired
- [ ] Bored
- [ ] Emotional

Hunger/Fullness scale:

Ravenous ●●●●● Stuffed

Protein

Carbs

Sugar

Fat

Calories

Sodium

Snack 3

I ate because I felt:
- [ ] Hungry
- [ ] Tired
- [ ] Bored
- [ ] Emotional

Hunger/Fullness scale:

Ravenous ●●●●● Stuffed

Protein

Carbs

Sugar

Fat

Calories

Sodium

Vitamins: Yes! [ ]   I forgot... [ ]

178

Daily Planner

Daily tasks:

♡ ....

♡ ....

♡ ....

♡ ....

♡ ....

My mood:

☹ ☹ 😐 🙂 😃

Hours of sleep:

2	3	4	5	6	7	8	9	10	11	12
☐	☐	☐	☐	☐	☐	☐	☐	☐	☐	☐

Today's affirmation:

....

....

Notes:

Daily schedule:

8.00	
9.00	
10.00	
11.00	
12.00	
1.00	
2.00	
3.00	
4.00	
5.00	
6.00	
7.00	
8.00	
9.00	
10.00	

179

Food Diary

Sunday _____

Breakfast

I ate because I felt:
- ☐ Hungry ☐ Bored
- ☐ Tired ☐ Emotional

Hunger/Fullness scale:

Ravenous ●●●●●○ Stuffed

Protein ○ Carbs ○ Sugar ○

Fat ○ Calories ○ Sodium ○

Lunch

I ate because I felt:
- ☐ Hungry ☐ Bored
- ☐ Tired ☐ Emotional

Hunger/Fullness scale:

Ravenous ●●●●●○ Stuffed

Protein ○ Carbs ○ Sugar ○

Fat ○ Calories ○ Sodium ○

Dinner

I ate because I felt:
- ☐ Hungry ☐ Bored
- ☐ Tired ☐ Emotional

Hunger/Fullness scale:

Ravenous ●●●●●○ Stuffed

Protein ○ Carbs ○ Sugar ○

Fat ○ Calories ○ Sodium ○

Snack 1

I ate because I felt:
- ☐ Hungry ☐ Bored
- ☐ Tired ☐ Emotional

Hunger/Fullness scale:

Ravenous ●●●●●○ Stuffed

Protein ○ Carbs ○ Sugar ○

Fat ○ Calories ○ Sodium ○

Snack 2

I ate because I felt:
- ☐ Hungry ☐ Bored
- ☐ Tired ☐ Emotional

Hunger/Fullness scale:

Ravenous ●●●●●○ Stuffed

Protein ○ Carbs ○ Sugar ○

Fat ○ Calories ○ Sodium ○

Snack 3

I ate because I felt:
- ☐ Hungry ☐ Bored
- ☐ Tired ☐ Emotional

Hunger/Fullness scale:

Ravenous ●●●●●○ Stuffed

Protein ○ Carbs ○ Sugar ○

Fat ○ Calories ○ Sodium ○

Vitamins: Yes! ☐ I forgot... ☐

Hydration Tracker Week 7

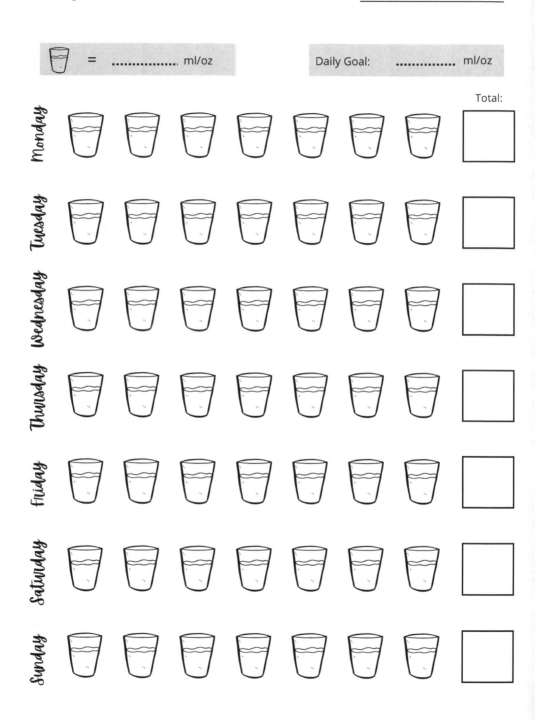

= .... ml/oz   Daily Goal: .... ml/oz

Total:

Monday

Tuesday

Wednesday

Thursday

friday

Saturday

Sunday

Meal Planner

Meals:

Grocery List:

Monday

Tuesday

Wednesday

Thursday

Friday

Saturday

Sunday

♡ ....
♡ ....
♡ ....
♡ ....
♡ ....
♡ ....
♡ ....
♡ ....
♡ ....
♡ ....
♡ ....
♡ ....
♡ ....
♡ ....
♡ ....
♡ ....
♡ ....
♡ ....
♡ ....
♡ ....

Activity Tracker

Week 7

Daily Target: .... minutes

Minutes:

Monday

Tuesday

Wednesday

Thursday

Friday

Saturday

Sunday

Habit Tracker

Habit	MON	TUE	WED	THU	FRI	SAT	SUN
	○	○	○	○	○	○	○
	○	○	○	○	○	○	○
	○	○	○	○	○	○	○
	○	○	○	○	○	○	○
	○	○	○	○	○	○	○
	○	○	○	○	○	○	○
	○	○	○	○	○	○	○
	○	○	○	○	○	○	○
	○	○	○	○	○	○	○
	○	○	○	○	○	○	○
	○	○	○	○	○	○	○
	○	○	○	○	○	○	○
	○	○	○	○	○	○	○
	○	○	○	○	○	○	○
	○	○	○	○	○	○	○
	○	○	○	○	○	○	○
	○	○	○	○	○	○	○

Notes:

Normalize different portion sizes after Bariatric Surgery.

You were never meant to eat 1 oz. of food forever.

Weigh-In

Highest Weight

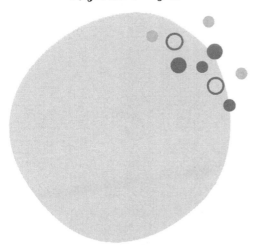

Weight Last Week

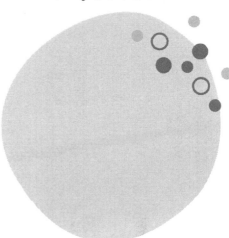

Weekly Weight Loss +/-

Current Weight

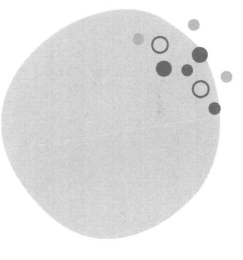

Notes:

Measurements

	Highest	Last Week	This Week	Lost
Neck				
Shoulders				
Chest				
Right Arm				
Left Arm				
Waist				
Hips				
Right Thigh				
Left Thigh				
Right Calf				
Left Calf				

Notes:

....

....

....

Progress Picture

Worthy Then   ## Worthy Now

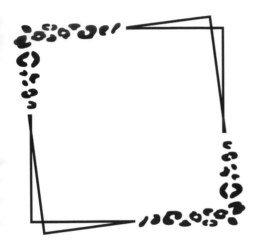   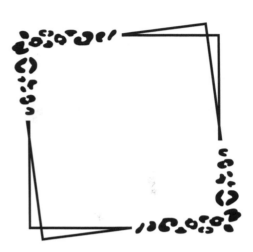

Date: ....   Date: ....

Weight: ....   Weight: ....

Describe how you felt in both pictures: _____

....

....

....

....

Reflection

Skills I have worked on this week:

....

....

....

....

I still need to be more mindful of:

....

....

....

....

I am thankful for:

....

....

....

....

Next week I will focus more on:

....

....

....

Brain Dump

What's on your mind?

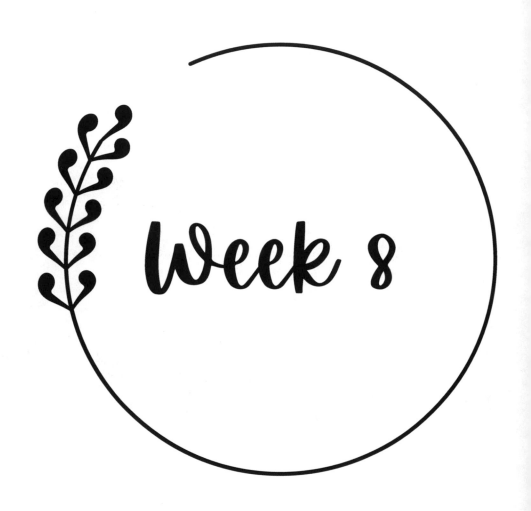

Week 8

Weekly Planner

Priorities:

♡ ....
♡ ....
♡ ....
♡ ....
♡ ....

To do:

☐ ....
☐ ....
☐ ....
☐ ....
☐ ....
☐ ....
☐ ....
☐ ....
☐ ....
☐ ....
☐ ....

Notes:

Monday

Tuesday

Wednesday

Thursday

Friday

Saturday

Sunday

Daily Planner

Daily tasks:

♡ ....
♡ ....
♡ ....
♡ ....
♡ ....

My mood:

☹ ☹ 😐 🙂 😃

Hours of sleep:

2 3 4 5 6 7 8 9 10 11 12
☐ ☐ ☐ ☐ ☐ ☐ ☐ ☐ ☐ ☐ ☐

Today's affirmation:

....

....

Notes:

Daily schedule:

8.00	
9.00	
10.00	
11.00	
12.00	
1.00	
2.00	
3.00	
4.00	
5.00	
6.00	
7.00	
8.00	
9.00	
10.00	

Food Diary

Breakfast

I ate because I felt:
- [ ] Hungry
- [ ] Tired
- [ ] Bored
- [ ] Emotional

Hunger/Fullness scale:

Ravenous · · · · · Stuffed

Protein Carbs Sugar

Fat Calories Sodium

Lunch

I ate because I felt:
- [ ] Hungry
- [ ] Tired
- [ ] Bored
- [ ] Emotional

Hunger/Fullness scale:

Ravenous · · · · · Stuffed

Protein Carbs Sugar

Fat Calories Sodium

Dinner

I ate because I felt:
- [ ] Hungry
- [ ] Tired
- [ ] Bored
- [ ] Emotional

Hunger/Fullness scale:

Ravenous · · · · · Stuffed

Protein Carbs Sugar

Fat Calories Sodium

Snack 1

I ate because I felt:
- [ ] Hungry
- [ ] Tired
- [ ] Bored
- [ ] Emotional

Hunger/Fullness scale:

Ravenous · · · · · Stuffed

Protein Carbs Sugar

Fat Calories Sodium

Snack 2

I ate because I felt:
- [ ] Hungry
- [ ] Tired
- [ ] Bored
- [ ] Emotional

Hunger/Fullness scale:

Ravenous · · · · · Stuffed

Protein Carbs Sugar

Fat Calories Sodium

Snack 3

I ate because I felt:
- [ ] Hungry
- [ ] Tired
- [ ] Bored
- [ ] Emotional

Hunger/Fullness scale:

Ravenous · · · · · Stuffed

Protein Carbs Sugar

Fat Calories Sodium

Vitamins: Yes! [ ] I forgot... [ ]

Daily Planner

Daily tasks:

♡ ....
♡ ....
♡ ....
♡ ....
♡ ....

My mood:

☹ ☹ 😐 🙂 😃

Hours of sleep:

2   3   4   5   6   7   8   9   10   11   12
☐ ☐ ☐ ☐ ☐ ☐ ☐ ☐   ☐   ☐   ☐

Today's affirmation:

....

....

Notes:

Daily schedule:

8.00	
9.00	
10.00	
11.00	
12.00	
1.00	
2.00	
3.00	
4.00	
5.00	
6.00	
7.00	
8.00	
9.00	
10.00	

Food Diary

Breakfast

I ate because I felt:

- [ ] Hungry
- [ ] Tired
- [ ] Bored
- [ ] Emotional

Hunger/Fullness scale:

Ravenous ●●●●●● Stuffed

Protein   Carbs   Sugar

Fat   Calories   Sodium

Lunch

I ate because I felt:

- [ ] Hungry
- [ ] Tired
- [ ] Bored
- [ ] Emotional

Hunger/Fullness scale:

Ravenous ●●●●●● Stuffed

Protein   Carbs   Sugar

Fat   Calories   Sodium

Dinner

I ate because I felt:

- [ ] Hungry
- [ ] Tired
- [ ] Bored
- [ ] Emotional

Hunger/Fullness scale:

Ravenous ●●●●●● Stuffed

Protein   Carbs   Sugar

Fat   Calories   Sodium

Snack 1

I ate because I felt:

- [ ] Hungry
- [ ] Tired
- [ ] Bored
- [ ] Emotional

Hunger/Fullness scale:

Ravenous ●●●●●● Stuffed

Protein   Carbs   Sugar

Fat   Calories   Sodium

Snack 2

I ate because I felt:

- [ ] Hungry
- [ ] Tired
- [ ] Bored
- [ ] Emotional

Hunger/Fullness scale:

Ravenous ●●●●●● Stuffed

Protein   Carbs   Sugar

Fat   Calories   Sodium

Snack 3

I ate because I felt:

- [ ] Hungry
- [ ] Tired
- [ ] Bored
- [ ] Emotional

Hunger/Fullness scale:

Ravenous ●●●●●● Stuffed

Protein   Carbs   Sugar

Fat   Calories   Sodium

Vitamins: Yes! [ ]   I forgot... [ ]

Daily Planner

Wednesday

Daily tasks:

♡ ....
♡ ....
♡ ....
♡ ....
♡ ....

My mood:

☹ ☹ 😐 🙂 😃

Hours of sleep:

2	3	4	5	6	7	8	9	10	11	12
☐	☐	☐	☐	☐	☐	☐	☐	☐	☐	☐

Today's affirmation:

....

....

Notes:

Daily schedule:

8.00	
9.00	
10.00	
11.00	
12.00	
1.00	
2.00	
3.00	
4.00	
5.00	
6.00	
7.00	
8.00	
9.00	
10.00	

Food Diary

Breakfast

I ate because I felt:

☐ Hungry ☐ Bored
☐ Tired ☐ Emotional

Hunger/Fullness scale:

Ravenous ● ● ● ● ● ○ Stuffed

Protein ○ Carbs ○ Sugar ○
Fat ○ Calories ○ Sodium ○

Lunch

I ate because I felt:

☐ Hungry ☐ Bored
☐ Tired ☐ Emotional

Hunger/Fullness scale:

Ravenous ● ● ● ● ● ○ Stuffed

Protein ○ Carbs ○ Sugar ○
Fat ○ Calories ○ Sodium ○

Dinner

I ate because I felt:

☐ Hungry ☐ Bored
☐ Tired ☐ Emotional

Hunger/Fullness scale:

Ravenous ● ● ● ● ● ○ Stuffed

Protein ○ Carbs ○ Sugar ○
Fat ○ Calories ○ Sodium ○

Snack 1

I ate because I felt:

☐ Hungry ☐ Bored
☐ Tired ☐ Emotional

Hunger/Fullness scale:

Ravenous ● ● ● ● ● ○ Stuffed

Protein ○ Carbs ○ Sugar ○
Fat ○ Calories ○ Sodium ○

Snack 2

I ate because I felt:

☐ Hungry ☐ Bored
☐ Tired ☐ Emotional

Hunger/Fullness scale:

Ravenous ● ● ● ● ● ○ Stuffed

Protein ○ Carbs ○ Sugar ○
Fat ○ Calories ○ Sodium ○

Snack 3

I ate because I felt:

☐ Hungry ☐ Bored
☐ Tired ☐ Emotional

Hunger/Fullness scale:

Ravenous ● ● ● ● ● ○ Stuffed

Protein ○ Carbs ○ Sugar ○
Fat ○ Calories ○ Sodium ○

Vitamins: Yes! ☐ I forgot... ☐

Daily Planner

Daily tasks:

♡ ....
♡ ....
♡ ....
♡ ....
♡ ....

My mood:

☹ ☹ 😐 ☺ 😃

Hours of sleep:

2	3	4	5	6	7	8	9	10	11	12
☐	☐	☐	☐	☐	☐	☐	☐	☐	☐	☐

Today's affirmation:

....

....

Notes:

Daily schedule:

8.00	
9.00	
10.00	
11.00	
12.00	
1.00	
2.00	
3.00	
4.00	
5.00	
6.00	
7.00	
8.00	
9.00	
10.00	

199

Food Diary

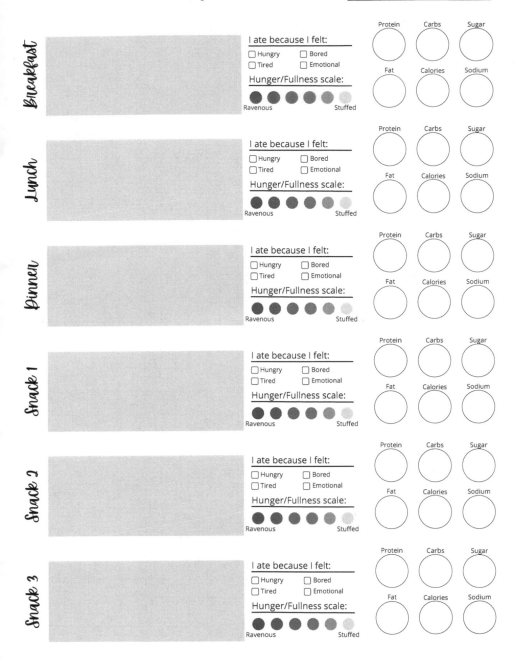

Breakfast

I ate because I felt:
- ☐ Hungry
- ☐ Bored
- ☐ Tired
- ☐ Emotional

Hunger/Fullness scale:

Ravenous ●●●●●● Stuffed

Protein   Carbs   Sugar

Fat   Calories   Sodium

Lunch

I ate because I felt:
- ☐ Hungry
- ☐ Bored
- ☐ Tired
- ☐ Emotional

Hunger/Fullness scale:

Ravenous ●●●●●● Stuffed

Protein   Carbs   Sugar

Fat   Calories   Sodium

Dinner

I ate because I felt:
- ☐ Hungry
- ☐ Bored
- ☐ Tired
- ☐ Emotional

Hunger/Fullness scale:

Ravenous ●●●●●● Stuffed

Protein   Carbs   Sugar

Fat   Calories   Sodium

Snack 1

I ate because I felt:
- ☐ Hungry
- ☐ Bored
- ☐ Tired
- ☐ Emotional

Hunger/Fullness scale:

Ravenous ●●●●●● Stuffed

Protein   Carbs   Sugar

Fat   Calories   Sodium

Snack 2

I ate because I felt:
- ☐ Hungry
- ☐ Bored
- ☐ Tired
- ☐ Emotional

Hunger/Fullness scale:

Ravenous ●●●●●● Stuffed

Protein   Carbs   Sugar

Fat   Calories   Sodium

Snack 3

I ate because I felt:
- ☐ Hungry
- ☐ Bored
- ☐ Tired
- ☐ Emotional

Hunger/Fullness scale:

Ravenous ●●●●●● Stuffed

Protein   Carbs   Sugar

Fat   Calories   Sodium

Vitamins: Yes! ☐   I forgot... ☐

Daily Planner

Friday

Daily tasks:

♡ ....
♡ ....
♡ ....
♡ ....
♡ ....

My mood:

☹ ☹ 😐 🙂 😄

Hours of sleep:

2 3 4 5 6 7 8 9 10 11 12
☐ ☐ ☐ ☐ ☐ ☐ ☐ ☐ ☐ ☐ ☐

Today's affirmation:

....
....

Notes:

Daily schedule:

8.00	
9.00	
10.00	
11.00	
12.00	
1.00	
2.00	
3.00	
4.00	
5.00	
6.00	
7.00	
8.00	
9.00	
10.00	

201

Food Diary

Friday _____

Breakfast

I ate because I felt:
- [ ] Hungry
- [ ] Tired
- [ ] Bored
- [ ] Emotional

Hunger/Fullness scale:

Ravenous ●●●●●● Stuffed

Protein | Carbs | Sugar

Fat | Calories | Sodium

Lunch

I ate because I felt:
- [ ] Hungry
- [ ] Tired
- [ ] Bored
- [ ] Emotional

Hunger/Fullness scale:

Ravenous ●●●●●● Stuffed

Protein | Carbs | Sugar

Fat | Calories | Sodium

Dinner

I ate because I felt:
- [ ] Hungry
- [ ] Tired
- [ ] Bored
- [ ] Emotional

Hunger/Fullness scale:

Ravenous ●●●●●● Stuffed

Protein | Carbs | Sugar

Fat | Calories | Sodium

Snack 1

I ate because I felt:
- [ ] Hungry
- [ ] Tired
- [ ] Bored
- [ ] Emotional

Hunger/Fullness scale:

Ravenous ●●●●●● Stuffed

Protein | Carbs | Sugar

Fat | Calories | Sodium

Snack 2

I ate because I felt:
- [ ] Hungry
- [ ] Tired
- [ ] Bored
- [ ] Emotional

Hunger/Fullness scale:

Ravenous ●●●●●● Stuffed

Protein | Carbs | Sugar

Fat | Calories | Sodium

Snack 3

I ate because I felt:
- [ ] Hungry
- [ ] Tired
- [ ] Bored
- [ ] Emotional

Hunger/Fullness scale:

Ravenous ●●●●●● Stuffed

Protein | Carbs | Sugar

Fat | Calories | Sodium

Vitamins: Yes! [ ]   I forgot... [ ]

202

Daily Planner

Daily tasks:

♡ ....

♡ ....

♡ ....

♡ ....

♡ ....

My mood:

☹ ☹ 😐 🙂 😃

Hours of sleep:

2 3 4 5 6 7 8 9 10 11 12
☐ ☐ ☐ ☐ ☐ ☐ ☐ ☐ ☐ ☐ ☐

Today's affirmation:

....

....

Notes:

Daily schedule:

8.00	
9.00	
10.00	
11.00	
12.00	
1.00	
2.00	
3.00	
4.00	
5.00	
6.00	
7.00	
8.00	
9.00	
10.00	

Food Diary

Saturday

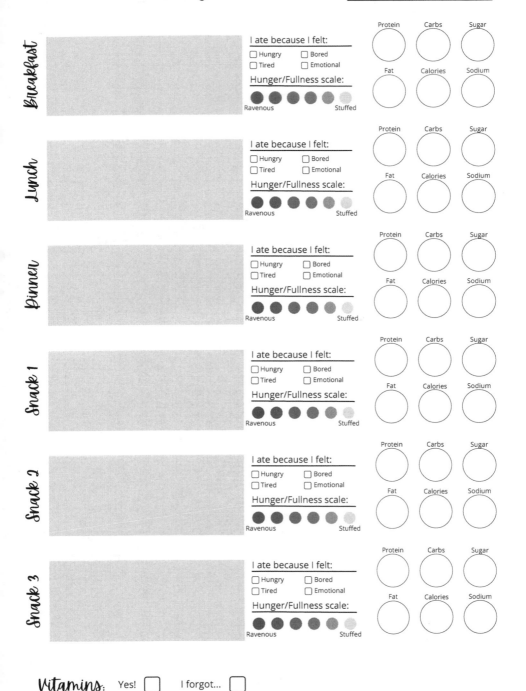

Breakfast

I ate because I felt:
- ☐ Hungry
- ☐ Bored
- ☐ Tired
- ☐ Emotional

Hunger/Fullness scale:

Ravenous ● ● ● ● ○ Stuffed

Protein / Carbs / Sugar

Fat / Calories / Sodium

Lunch

I ate because I felt:
- ☐ Hungry
- ☐ Bored
- ☐ Tired
- ☐ Emotional

Hunger/Fullness scale:

Ravenous ● ● ● ● ○ Stuffed

Protein / Carbs / Sugar

Fat / Calories / Sodium

Dinner

I ate because I felt:
- ☐ Hungry
- ☐ Bored
- ☐ Tired
- ☐ Emotional

Hunger/Fullness scale:

Ravenous ● ● ● ● ○ Stuffed

Protein / Carbs / Sugar

Fat / Calories / Sodium

Snack 1

I ate because I felt:
- ☐ Hungry
- ☐ Bored
- ☐ Tired
- ☐ Emotional

Hunger/Fullness scale:

Ravenous ● ● ● ● ○ Stuffed

Protein / Carbs / Sugar

Fat / Calories / Sodium

Snack 2

I ate because I felt:
- ☐ Hungry
- ☐ Bored
- ☐ Tired
- ☐ Emotional

Hunger/Fullness scale:

Ravenous ● ● ● ● ○ Stuffed

Protein / Carbs / Sugar

Fat / Calories / Sodium

Snack 3

I ate because I felt:
- ☐ Hungry
- ☐ Bored
- ☐ Tired
- ☐ Emotional

Hunger/Fullness scale:

Ravenous ● ● ● ● ○ Stuffed

Protein / Carbs / Sugar

Fat / Calories / Sodium

Vitamins: Yes! ☐   I forgot... ☐

Daily Planner

Daily tasks:

♡ ....
♡ ....
♡ ....
♡ ....
♡ ....

My mood:

☹ ☹ 😐 🙂 😃

Hours of sleep:

2	3	4	5	6	7	8	9	10	11	12
☐	☐	☐	☐	☐	☐	☐	☐	☐	☐	☐

Today's affirmation:

....

....

Notes:

Daily schedule:

Time	
8.00	
9.00	
10.00	
11.00	
12.00	
1.00	
2.00	
3.00	
4.00	
5.00	
6.00	
7.00	
8.00	
9.00	
10.00	

Food Diary

Breakfast

I ate because I felt:
- ☐ Hungry
- ☐ Tired
- ☐ Bored
- ☐ Emotional

Hunger/Fullness scale:

Ravenous ●●●●●○ Stuffed

Protein | Carbs | Sugar

Fat | Calories | Sodium

Lunch

I ate because I felt:
- ☐ Hungry
- ☐ Tired
- ☐ Bored
- ☐ Emotional

Hunger/Fullness scale:

Ravenous ●●●●●○ Stuffed

Protein | Carbs | Sugar

Fat | Calories | Sodium

Dinner

I ate because I felt:
- ☐ Hungry
- ☐ Tired
- ☐ Bored
- ☐ Emotional

Hunger/Fullness scale:

Ravenous ●●●●●○ Stuffed

Protein | Carbs | Sugar

Fat | Calories | Sodium

Snack 1

I ate because I felt:
- ☐ Hungry
- ☐ Tired
- ☐ Bored
- ☐ Emotional

Hunger/Fullness scale:

Ravenous ●●●●●○ Stuffed

Protein | Carbs | Sugar

Fat | Calories | Sodium

Snack 2

I ate because I felt:
- ☐ Hungry
- ☐ Tired
- ☐ Bored
- ☐ Emotional

Hunger/Fullness scale:

Ravenous ●●●●●○ Stuffed

Protein | Carbs | Sugar

Fat | Calories | Sodium

Snack 3

I ate because I felt:
- ☐ Hungry
- ☐ Tired
- ☐ Bored
- ☐ Emotional

Hunger/Fullness scale:

Ravenous ●●●●●○ Stuffed

Protein | Carbs | Sugar

Fat | Calories | Sodium

Vitamins: Yes! ☐   I forgot... ☐

Hydration Tracker Week 8

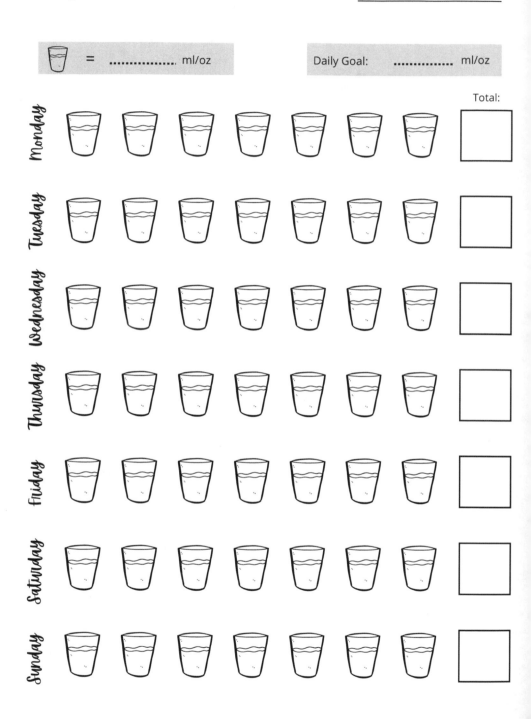

Meal Planner

Week 8

Meals:

Grocery List:

Monday	
Tuesday	
Wednesday	
Thursday	
Friday	
Saturday	
Sunday	

♡ ....
♡ ....
♡ ....
♡ ....
♡ ....
♡ ....
♡ ....
♡ ....
♡ ....
♡ ....
♡ ....
♡ ....
♡ ....
♡ ....
♡ ....
♡ ....
♡ ....
♡ ....
♡ ....
♡ ....
♡ ....
♡ ....
♡ ....
♡ ....

Activity Tracker

Week 8

Daily Target: .... minutes

Minutes:

Monday

Tuesday

Wednesday

Thursday

Friday

Saturday

Sunday

Habit Tracker

Habit	MON	TUE	WED	THU	FRI	SAT	SUN
	○	○	○	○	○	○	○
	○	○	○	○	○	○	○
	○	○	○	○	○	○	○
	○	○	○	○	○	○	○
	○	○	○	○	○	○	○
	○	○	○	○	○	○	○
	○	○	○	○	○	○	○
	○	○	○	○	○	○	○
	○	○	○	○	○	○	○
	○	○	○	○	○	○	○
	○	○	○	○	○	○	○
	○	○	○	○	○	○	○
	○	○	○	○	○	○	○
	○	○	○	○	○	○	○
	○	○	○	○	○	○	○
	○	○	○	○	○	○	○
	○	○	○	○	○	○	○

Notes:

True healing after Bariatric Surgery goes way beyond the mending of your incisions.

Weigh-In

Highest Weight

Weight Last Week

Weekly Weight Loss +/-

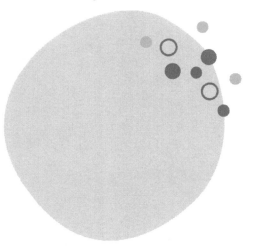

Current Weight

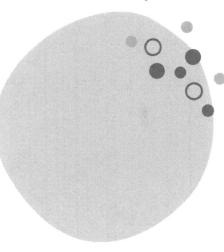

Notes:

212

Measurements

	Highest	Last Week	This Week	Lost
Neck				
Shoulders				
Chest				
Right Arm				
Left Arm				
Waist				
Hips				
Right Thigh				
Left Thigh				
Right Calf				
Left Calf				

Notes:

....

....

....

Progress Picture

Worthy Then

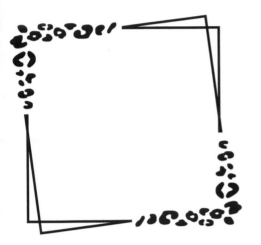

Worthy Now

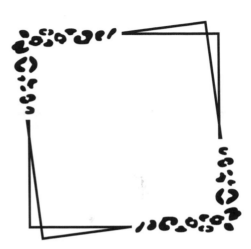

Date: ....

Weight: ....

Date: ....

Weight: ....

Describe how you felt in both pictures:

....

....

....

....

Reflection

Skills I have worked on this week:

....

....

....

....

I still need to be more mindful of:

....

....

....

....

I am thankful for:

....

....

....

....

Next week I will focus more on:

....

....

....

Brain Dump

What's on your mind?

Bonus - Colorful Weight Loss

Color the hearts for every pound or kilogram lost

Bonus - Colorful Weight Loss

Color the hearts for every pound or kilogram lost

Notes

Notes

Notes

Notes

Made in the USA
Middletown, DE
03 October 2022